Fast Facts:
Glaucoma

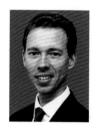

Paul R Healey MBBS(Hons) BMedSc(Cell Biol)
MMed(Clin Epidemiol) PhD(Med) FRANZCO
Clinical Senior Lecturer
University of Sydney
Department of Ophthalmology
Centre for Vision Research
Westmead Millennium Institute & Save Sight Institute
New South Wales, Australia

Glaucoma Specialist
Eye Associates
Sydney, Australia

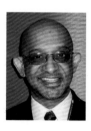

Ravi Thomas MBBS MD FRANZCO
Director of Glaucoma Services
Queensland Eye Institute and
Professor, University of Queensland
Brisbane, Australia

Previously:
Professor & Head, Department of Ophthalmology
Christian Medical College, Vellore, India
Director, LV Prasad Eye Institute
Banjara Hills, Hyderabad, Andhra Pradesh, India

Declaration of Independence
This book is as balanced and as practical as we can make it.
Ideas for improvement are always welcome: feedback@fastfacts.com

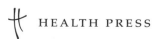
HEALTH PRESS

Fast Facts: Glaucoma
First published March 2010

Health Press Limited, Elizabeth House, Queen Street, Abingdon,
Oxford OX14 3LN, UK
Tel: +44 (0)1235 523233
Fax: +44 (0)1235 523238

Book orders can be placed by telephone or via the website.
For regional distributors or to order via the website, please go to:
www.fastfacts.com

For telephone orders, please call +44 (0)1752 202301 (UK and Europe),
1 800 247 6553 (USA, toll free), +1 419 281 1802 (Americas) or
+61 (0)2 9698 7755 (Asia–Pacific).

Fast Facts is a trademark of Health Press Limited.

A CIP record for this title is available from the British Library.

ISBN 978-1-905832-40-8

Healey PR (Paul)
Fast Facts: Glaucoma/
Paul R Healey, Ravi Thomas

Cover: Glaucoma is an increased pressure in the eyeball due to an excessive amount
of aqueous humour (the fluid that fills the eyeball). Seen here are the blood vessels
(red) and the optic disc (yellow), which is raised with a central bulge or 'cup' (white).
David Mack/Science Photo Library

Medical illustrations by Dee McLean, London, UK.
Typesetting and page layout by Zed, Oxford, UK.
Printed by Latimer Trend and Company Limited, Plymouth, UK.

Text printed on biodegradable and recyclable paper
manufactured using elemental chlorine free (ECF)
wood pulp from well-managed forests.

FSC
Mixed Sources
Product group from well-managed
forests and other controlled sources
Cert no. SGS-COC-005493
www.fsc.org
© 1996 Forest Stewardship Council

Glossary

Amblyopia: a decrease in vision for which no cause can be found on examination; in appropriate cases, amblyopia is correctable by therapeutic measures

(Primary) angle closure: obstruction of the trabecular meshwork by the iris in the absence of any detectable preceding causative disease

Angle-closure glaucoma: glaucomatous optic neuropathy due to raised IOP caused by obstruction of the iridocorneal angle by the iris

CDR: (optic) cup-to-disc ratio

Cyclophotocoagulation: procedure to destroy the ciliary processes, usually performed with a diode laser

Cycloplegic agent: topical drops used to paralyse the ciliary muscle; they also dilate the pupil

Fundus: the inner part of the eye visualized on ophthalmoscopy (fundoscopy): optic disc, retina, macula, blood vessels, etc.

Hypermetropia: condition of the eye where, with the accommodation at rest, parallel rays of light focus at a point behind the retina, usually because the axial length of the eyeball is smaller than normal

Hypotony: a syndrome of reduced vision and/or retinal swelling or folds caused by a very low eye pressure

IOP: intraocular pressure

Iridocorneal angle: the angle created by the junction of the cornea and iris; the outflow channels for aqueous drainage (trabecular meshwork) are located here

Lamina cribrosa: a sieve-like structure in the optic nerve head through which nerve fibers from the retina pass; blood vessels enter and leave the eye through this structure

Myopia: condition of the eye where, with the accommodation at rest, parallel rays of light focus at a point in front of the retina, usually because the axial length of the eyeball is larger than normal

Neuroretinal rim: the area of the optic disc occupied by the axons of the optic nerve (the 'left over' space is the cup)

Neuroretinal rim notch: a focal area of loss of the neuroretinal rim; notches are often seen in glaucoma

Open-angle glaucoma: glaucoma in the presence of anatomically normal iridocorneal angle structures, as seen on gonioscopy

Optic cup: the space left over in the optic disc after accommodating the retinal axons that form the optic nerve

Optic disc: the region of the fundus where the axons aggregate to form the optic nerve and exit the eye

PAS: peripheral anterior synechiae; an adhesion of the iris to the iridocorneal angle

PGA: prostaglandin analog

Primary angle-closure suspect: a patient whose angles are at risk of closure but who has no structural or functional signs of the disease

Primary glaucoma: glaucoma with no detectable preceding causative disease

Relative afferent pupillary defect (RAPD): an abnormal response in which one pupil dilates, rather than constricts, when a light is shone alternately on it and the other eye

Scotoma: a visual-field defect

Secondary exotropia: an outward deviation of the eye due to loss of vision

Secondary glaucoma: glaucoma with an identifiable cause of angle damage

Tonometry: measurement of the pressure within the eye

Trabecular meshwork: mesh-like structure at the iridoscleral angle, which allows aqueous humor to flow from the eye

Vascular dysregulation: a condition in which blood flow is not properly distributed to meet the demands of different tissues (includes Raynaud's phenomenon)

Introduction

Glaucoma is a chronic neurodegenerative disease of the optic nerve (the second cranial nerve). It is the most common neurodegenerative disease, affecting about 70 million people worldwide. Glaucoma is the second most common disease causing blindness after cataract, although the speed and degree of vision loss vary. Glaucoma blindness is irreversible but preventable. However, most people with glaucoma are not diagnosed or treated.

As yet, we have no tests that show the pathogenic mechanism at work in glaucoma. So, clinically, the disease is diagnosed and treated as a syndrome. Unfortunately, symptoms do not usually become noticeable until the late stages of glaucoma, because of neural compensation mechanisms. Nevertheless, quality of life can still be impaired relatively early in the course of the disease.

Clinical diagnosis consists of identifying the signs of structural damage in the eye (spatially localized loss of ganglion cells on the retina and at the optic disc) with matching loss of function (reduction in differential light sensitivity or amplitude of visual evoked potentials in the corresponding part of the visual field).

A number of risk factors for the onset and progression of glaucoma have been identified, of which raised intraocular pressure (IOP) is the most important. Corticosteroid use and contact between the iris and trabecular meshwork (angle closure) are modifiable risk factors for glaucoma, which act via raised IOP. Cardiovascular disease (including high and low blood pressure) is also a risk factor, acting via both raised IOP and possibly reduced perfusion of the optic nerve.

Treatment of glaucoma is based on reducing risk factors (almost always IOP) and improving quality of life. Lowering the IOP is a generic strategy for protecting the optic nerve, even when the initial IOP is not particularly high. The aim is to keep the IOP at a level at which disease progression is anticipated to be at an acceptably low rate. Medicines that may protect the visual pathways at a cellular level are being researched and developed, but no treatment can regenerate the optic nerve.

The management of glaucoma requires life-long monitoring for risk factors and checking optic nerve structure and function to determine whether the risk or disease state has changed. Results can be fed back into a management plan and the desired (target) IOP revised where necessary.

The diagnosis and treatment of glaucoma is made difficult by a number of factors.

- Visual disability often does not become apparent until the patient is almost blind.
- The 'normal' appearance of the optic disc varies enormously, making early diagnosis of structural damage difficult.
- Accurate measurement of vision loss from glaucoma requires expensive visual field analyzers and training for the clinician and their staff. False positive visual field test results are common in inexperienced patients.
- Risk factors for glaucoma in the absence of glaucomatous optic neuropathy are usually not sufficient to warrant prophylactic treatment (with the exception of a very high IOP or angle closure).
- The degree of IOP lowering required to stabilize glaucoma is different for each patient.
- Worsening of glaucoma usually occurs over years, making change difficult to recognize.
- Lowering the eye pressure surgically is challenging.
- We do not fully understand how glaucoma occurs, and have no treatments to directly prevent or cure it.

The aim of *Fast Facts: Glaucoma* is to provide a clear understanding of glaucoma: what it is, how to detect it and how to treat it. We hope this book will serve as a ready reference for all medical and eyecare practitioners, an aid for students and scientists involved in the study of eye disease and a sound overview for anyone interested in this challenging disease.

Several well-conducted population-based studies have investigated the prevalence and incidence of glaucoma and the risk factors associated with the disease. Additional information about risk factors and the natural history of glaucoma has been gleaned from well-conducted randomized controlled trials of treatment.

Definitions

Because it is diagnosed as a syndrome, the frequency (prevalence) of glaucoma varies depending on how it is defined. As the condition develops slowly, most definitions come from cross-sectional studies. Loose definitions are based on either the appearance of the optic nerve head or a visual field defect that is typical in glaucoma. The perceived influence of intraocular pressure (IOP) has been so strong that some (mostly older) studies defined glaucoma as any eye with a pressure above the normal range (8–21 mmHg for most populations), even in the absence of any detectable nerve damage.

Stricter (more modern) definitions of glaucoma require correlation between structural damage at the optic disc and functional abnormalities of the visual field typical of glaucoma, or an amount of nerve tissue in the optic nerve head that is less than the extreme end of the normal population distribution (i.e. 97.5th or 99th percentile). This is based on the assumption that the smaller the area of nerve tissue in the optic nerve head, the more likely it is to have been destroyed by glaucoma. In longitudinal studies glaucoma is defined as either the loss of tissue from the neuroretinal rim of the optic nerve head or the new development of a reproducible visual field defect that is typical of glaucoma. The 'typical' findings of glaucoma are summarized in Table 1.1.

Subtypes of glaucoma

Because IOP is such an important modifiable risk factor for glaucoma, subtypes of glaucoma are classified according to the cause or mechanism

TABLE 1.1

Findings 'typical' of glaucoma

No one sign is diagnostic. There are no standardized criteria for diagnosis, but a combination of signs provides the strongest indicator, particularly when structural and functional signs match.

Structural signs – loss of optic nerve tissue within the eye

- Neuroretinal rim notch – focal (usually lower or upper) thinning or a complete absence of the rim of the optic nerve

- Large cup-to-disc ratio – generalized loss of neuroretinal rim tissue manifesting as a large optic cup compared with the size of the optic disc

- Focal or generalized defects (loss) of the retinal nerve fiber layer

Functional symptoms – decreased optic nerve function in visual field locations that correspond to structural damage

- Focal visual field defects (scotomas) that appear to arise from the blind spot (the position of the optic nerve head in the visual field) but do not cross the horizontal midline

- Scotomas can occur in isolation or in combination in the nasal, paracentral or peripheral parts of the upper or lower hemifields

- Coalescence of scotomas with loss of central vision but retention of temporal visual field (in advanced glaucoma)

of the increased IOP, which usually means the mechanism of damage to the aqueous outflow pathways of the eye. Figure 1.1 shows the two pathways through which aqueous fluid leaves the eye: the trabecular and uveoscleral outflow pathways. Aqueous production from the cells lining the ciliary body does not increase in eyes with high IOP. The uveoscleral pathway usually drains only a small proportion of aqueous. The main determinant of IOP is the resistance to flow through the trabecular meshwork; diseases that damage the trabecular outflow pathway frequently raise IOP.

It is important to remember that the subtypes, as shown in Figure 1.2, refer to the different causes of raised IOP, not to different types of optic neuropathy. Glaucomatous optic neuropathy – which

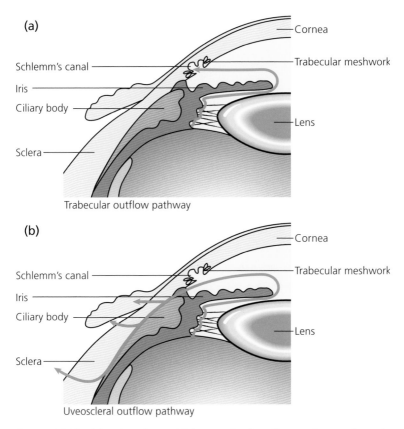

Figure 1.1 The (a) trabecular and (b) uveoscleral outflow pathways through which aqueous fluid leaves the eye.

appears to be fundamentally the same for all types of glaucoma – depends on the balance between risk factors and protective factors, rather than the cause of the risk factor.

Primary glaucomas are diseases that have no detectable preceding causative disease.

Primary open-angle glaucoma (OAG). In primary OAG there is no visible damage or blockage in the iridocorneal angle where the trabecular outflow pathway lies (see Figure 1.1). The IOP in primary OAG can vary from extremely high to the low end of the normal range. Some clinicians use the term 'normal tension glaucoma' to denote OAG

11

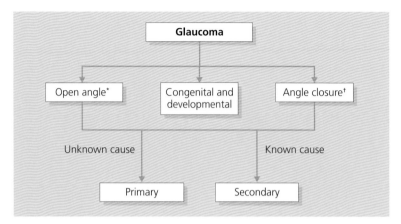

Figure 1.2 Subtypes of glaucoma. *Also called chronic glaucoma. 'Normal tension glaucoma' is defined as open-angle glaucoma with intraocular pressure in the population normal range. [†]Also called acute, closed-angle, narrow-angle glaucoma.

where the presenting IOP is within the population normal range. There are two possible explanations as to why the IOP in OAG is so variable. There may be a subset of OAG where damage is independent of IOP. Alternatively, the susceptibility of the optic nerve head to the effects of pressure may vary greatly; for some eyes, even a low IOP can be too high.

Primary angle-closure glaucoma (ACG), the other main subtype of primary glaucoma, is caused by raised IOP resulting from blockage of the trabecular outflow pathway by the iris. As the iris blocks the trabecular meshwork, the iridocorneal angle becomes closed and the IOP rises to high levels. Primary ACG is always associated with a narrow space between the iris and the trabecular meshwork, hence its historical names of narrow-angle or closed-angle glaucoma. ACG is always preceded by primary angle closure, where the angle is partly closed and the IOP may be elevated but the optic nerve has not yet sustained damage. While the underlying cause of the primary angle closure is unknown, the wide variation between populations suggests a genetic basis.

Developmental glaucomas. Congenital glaucoma is the most frequent developmental glaucoma, in which high IOP is caused by a genetic maldevelopment of the outflow pathway structures in the iridocorneal angle. The most common genetic associations are abnormalities in the *CYP1B1* gene that encodes cytochrome P450 1B1. Congenital glaucoma is present at or before birth. In other developmental glaucomas, genetic abnormalities damage the outflow pathway structures causing a severe increase in IOP early in life. Some developmental glaucomas have been linked to specific gene defects.

Secondary glaucomas. In secondary glaucoma, an identifiable disease causes secondary angle damage.

Pseudoexfoliation syndrome is by far the most common secondary glaucoma syndrome. In this syndrome a genetic abnormality of elastin causes a build up of material on and in the trabecular meshwork and a rise in IOP in about half of affected eyes. Although associated with a variant of the *LOXL1* gene, pseudoexfoliation syndrome is detected clinically and so can be missed early in the disease. For this reason, pseudoexfoliation glaucoma is usually included with primary OAG in clinical and epidemiological studies.

Pigment dispersion syndrome is a rarer secondary OAG caused by abnormal shedding of melanin pigment from the iris, which results in blockage of the trabecular meshwork.

Other secondary glaucomas include OAG caused by corticosteroids (which induce a decrease in trabecular outflow facility), trabecular injury from eye trauma, inflammation (uveitis), blood, or lens particles from advanced cataract. Secondary ACG may occur where the iris is either pulled onto the trabecular meshwork by ischemic neovascularization (e.g. from diabetes or a retinal vein occlusion) or pushed there by a very large lens or anterior rotation of the ciliary body.

Prevalence of glaucoma subtypes

The worldwide prevalence of glaucoma varies by geographic region (Figure 1.3). The prevalence of glaucoma increases exponentially with age; thus, variations in the aged population explain much of the variation in glaucoma. The exceptions are some parts of Africa (and to a lesser extent Latin America and Japan), where the prevalence of OAG is increased despite a younger population, and in China/South East Asia

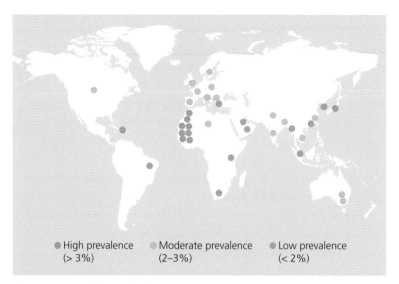

Figure 1.3 Prevalence of glaucoma in people over 40 years of age by geographic region. Prevalence in the USA varies with ethnicity but in general is moderate.

and India where rates of ACG are much higher than in other parts of the world.

Primary open-angle glaucoma (including pseudoexfoliation glaucoma) is the most common type of glaucoma in all regions worldwide. Estimates of prevalence vary between 1% and 4% of the population over 40 years of age. Approximately 45 million people have OAG.

By ethnicity. The frequency of OAG is highest in West African and emigrant populations (7–9%). Rates in other African, European and Asian populations lie between 1% and 2%; prevalence is about 3.2% in Japan and South America. Japan is unusual in that the majority of people with glaucoma have IOP within the normal population range (known as normal tension glaucoma).

By age. The prevalence of OAG rises dramatically with increasing age: as can be seen from Figure 1.4, the rate can be as high as 20% of the population over 80 years of age. With worldwide life expectancy increasing enormously this century, glaucoma is destined to become a much more common eye disease.

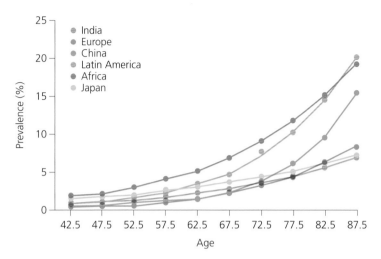

Figure 1.4 The age-specific prevalence of open-angle glaucoma from a number of epidemiological studies in different regions of the world. Prevalence is highest among the African and Latin American groups. Reproduced with permission from Quigley HA, Broman AT. The number of people with glaucoma worldwide in 2010 and 2020. *Br J Ophthalmol* 2006;90:262–7.

By IOP. Most population-based studies suggest that 30–70% of people with OAG have IOP within the normal range. In Japan, this figure is as high as 92%.

Primary angle-closure glaucoma is only one-third as common as OAG, but the regional prevalence of ACG varies greatly. Combined with the more severe natural history, ACG is a disproportionately high cause of glaucoma blindness worldwide. Historically, ACG was thought to be extremely rare and always to manifest with acute symptoms due to very high IOP. This very painful condition was called 'acute angle-closure glaucoma' but, because there was often no glaucomatous damage at the time of presentation, it has been simplified to 'acute angle closure'. Epidemiological studies now suggest that most ACG is caused by asymptomatic chronic angle closure (CAC).

By ethnicity. ACG is found in all populations but is much more common amongst the Inuit (2.65%), Mongolian, and resident and emigrant Chinese populations (about 1.5%) than in Europeans (0.1–0.2%). The prevalence in Indian populations is between 0.1% and 2.65%. Angle closure and ACG are important public health problems in the very large Chinese and Indian populations. Indeed, in China the rate of ACG almost parallels that of OAG, but the former causes more blindness.

By age. The prevalence of ACG increases with age in a similar manner to OAG, although the highest age-specific prevalence estimates are still much lower than for OAG – about 5% of the population. This is partly counterbalanced by the higher rate of blindness in ACG.

Congenital glaucoma is present at birth and most cases are diagnosed during the first year of life, although sometimes symptoms are not recognized until later in infancy or early childhood. Congenital glaucoma is rare in most populations: rates range from 2.85 cases per 100000 births in Spain, to 4.5 per 100000 births in Slovakia. However, populations with a high prevalence of the underlying genetic mutation have much higher rates of primary congenital glaucoma (e.g. 80 per 100000 in Slovakian gypsies and high rates in some middle-eastern populations).

Pediatric glaucomas are rarer than congenital glaucomas and are more diverse in etiology, although they are also usually genetic. Infantile glaucomas present within the first 3 years of life, and juvenile glaucomas after this. They are characterized by very high IOPs. Some are associated with other developmental syndromes, and specific genetic defects have been identified for some.

Secondary glaucoma. Rates of secondary glaucoma depend on the rates of the underlying causes (see above), but generally this condition is found in 0.1–0.5% of the adult population over 40 years of age.

Incidence
As glaucoma is a chronic disease for which there is no cure, individuals have the disease for life. The incidence of OAG varies from 0.5 to 1.1%

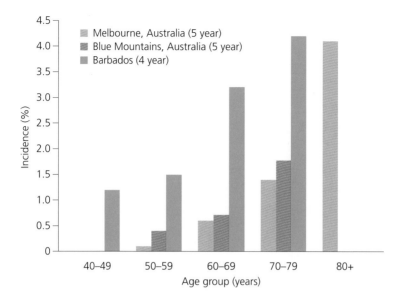

Figure 1.5 The age-specific incidence of open-angle glaucoma from a number of epidemiological studies in Australia and Barbados, showing a steep increase in incidence with age.

over 5 years, and 4.5% over 10 years in European-derived populations. In populations derived from West Africa, incidences of 2.2% over 4 years and 8.5% over 9 years have been reported. The incidence of glaucoma increases steeply with age (Figure 1.5).

Blindness

Glaucoma is the most common cause of irreversible blindness. Worldwide modeling suggests that in 2010 4.5 million people will be bilaterally blind from OAG and 4 million from ACG. While rates of OAG are higher than ACG everywhere, primary ACG more frequently causes blindness because of the very high IOPs and its high prevalence in the developing world. This is also why glaucoma causes more blindness in Asia than in other regions of the world. Predictions suggest that by 2020, over 11 million people will be bilaterally blind from glaucoma.

Secondary glaucoma also frequently causes blindness, but it is usually unilateral, so the overall effect on vision is less.

TABLE 1.2

Risk factors for glaucoma

Risk factor	Glaucoma type	Strength of risk	Strength of evidence	Type of study
Systemic				
Older age	OAG	+++	Excellent	ES, RCT
	ACG	+	Good	ES
Female sex	ACG	++	Good	ES
Family history	OAG	+	Fair	ES
BP abnormalities	OAG	+	Modest	ES, RCT
Ocular				
Higher intraocular pressure	All*	+++	Excellent	ES, RCT
Optic disc hemorrhage	OAG	+++	Good	ES, RCT
Pseudoexfoliation syndrome	OAG	++	Good	RCT, ES
Myopia	OAG	+	Fair	ES
Thinner central cornea	OAG	+	Fair	ES, RCT
Narrow iridocorneal angle	ACG	+	Good	ES
Disease state				
Angle closure	ACG	+++	Good	ES
More severe field loss	OAG	+	Fair	RCT
Bilateral vision loss	OAG	+	Modest	RCT
Less nerve tissue (larger CDR)	OAG	+	Modest	RCT, ES

+++, very strong; ++, strong; +, moderate. *Includes normal tension glaucoma.
ACG, angle-closure glaucoma; BP, blood pressure; CDR, cup-to-disc ratio;
ES, epidemiological study; OAG, open-angle glaucoma; RCT, randomized
controlled trial.

Congenital and pediatric glaucomas cause a large burden of disability in terms of both visual impairment during the prime of life and the requirement for lifelong follow-up.

Risk factors

Both epidemiological studies and randomized controlled trials have identified risk factors for OAG. Risk factors for ACG are less well documented (apart from angle closure itself) (Table 1.2).

Family history. About 60% of people with glaucoma have a relative with the disease. First-degree relatives of individuals with OAG have a three- to eightfold increased risk of glaucoma (compared with those with no family history of the disease). Less information is available concerning ACG.

Key points – definitions and epidemiology

- Glaucoma is diagnosed as a syndrome.
- Diagnosis is based on observing loss of optic nerve fibers leading to characteristic optic nerve changes within the eye and corresponding defects in the visual field.
- Glaucoma is classified on the basis of intraocular pressure risk factors.
- The main subtypes are primary and secondary types of open-angle and angle-closure glaucoma and developmental glaucomas.
- The prevalence of glaucoma varies between 1% and 8% of people over 40 years of age.
- Rates of angle-closure glaucoma vary more widely and account for proportionally more blindness.
- Glaucoma prevalence and incidence increases greatly with increasing age and is much more common among family members of those affected.

Cell damage

The pathophysiology of glaucoma is not fully understood. Vision loss in glaucoma is caused by damage to retinal ganglion cells. These are the last cells in the eye's visual neural network, which begins with the photoreceptors (rods and cones) and terminates with the retinal ganglion cells, the axons of which synapse in the lateral geniculate nucleus in the thalamus (Figure 2.1). The pattern of damage to the retinal ganglion cells in glaucoma suggests that the primary site of injury is the optic nerve head, the region where ganglion cells coalesce and turn through the optic disc to exit the eye. In eyes with glaucoma and high intraocular pressure (IOP) there is posterior bowing and compression of the lamina cribrosa (a sieve-like extension of the sclera in the optic nerve head through which nerve fibers from the retina pass, and through

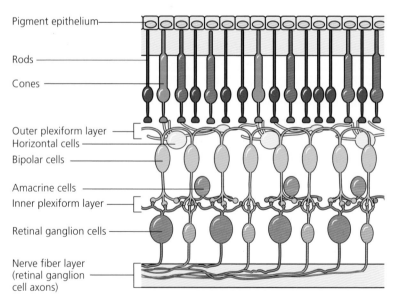

Pigment epithelium

Rods

Cones

Outer plexiform layer
Horizontal cells
Bipolar cells

Amacrine cells
Inner plexiform layer

Retinal ganglion cells

Nerve fiber layer
(retinal ganglion
cell axons)

Figure 2.1 Damage in glaucoma occurs principally to the retinal ganglion cells, the last cells in the neural network, which begins with the photoreceptors and terminates at the optic nerve in the lateral geniculate nucleus in the thalamus.

which blood vessels enter and leave the eye). This compression is associated with the characteristic structural loss at the neuroretinal rim of the optic disc – a clinical characteristic called 'cupping' because of the secondary enlargement of the optic cup (Figure 2.2).

Laboratory studies suggest that the death of ganglion cells in glaucoma is primarily by apoptosis. Apoptosis is an orderly process of self-destruction that requires activation of a number of intracellular pathways. The roles of the various extrinsic and intrinsic pathways that lead to the apoptotic cascade in glaucoma are being investigated.

Before apoptosis, retinal ganglion cells may undergo reversible structural and functional changes, such as reduced cell and axon size, dendritic arborization and neurofilament production. In addition, they may produce neuroprotective substances such as heat shock proteins.

The death of ganglion cells causes secondary (apoptotic) degeneration of the connected neurons of the optic tract, which connect the lateral geniculate nucleus to the primary visual cortex. Other retinal neurons (photoreceptors, bipolar cells) and the visual cortex neurons do not appear to be affected by glaucoma.

Support cells in the retina and optic nerve such as Müller cells and astrocytes may be damaged in glaucoma. Dysfunction in these cells has been postulated to be the primary insult in glaucoma, either by loss of normal protective function or decompensatory release of ganglion cell toxins. Astrocytes in the optic nerve head react to fluctuations in IOP and probably regulate the strength and compliance of the lamina cribrosa, through which the retinal ganglion cells pass to form the optic nerve. Loss of this function may render the ganglion cells susceptible to blockage of axoplasmic flow and deprive them of vital substances such as brain-derived neurotrophic factor from the other end of the cell. Astrocytes may also produce toxins such as nitric oxide. Retinal Müller cells play an important role in sequestration of excitotoxic neurotransmitters such as glutamate. Loss of this function could lead to the death of ganglion cells by excitotoxicity.

A normal retina has between 800 000 and 1 200 000 ganglion cells, and approximately twice this number before birth. It is thought that fetal ganglion cells that do not make cerebral synapses die by apoptosis. Ganglion cells are lost normally throughout life – about 25% of cells are lost over a 75-year life span.

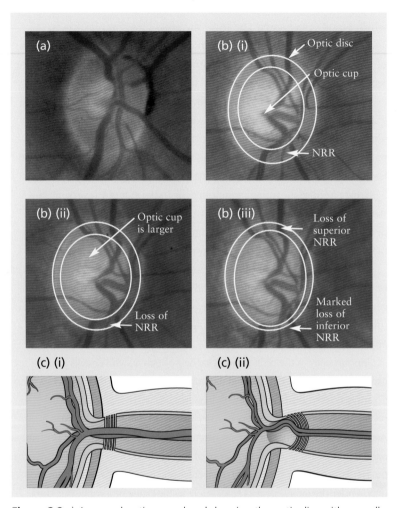

Figure 2.2 a) A normal optic nerve head showing the optic disc with a small optic cup in the center. The ganglion cells lie at the neuroretinal rim (NRR) of the optic disc. The lamina cribrosa, which extends beneath the neural tissue, can be seen at the base of the cup. b) Optic nerve damage from glaucoma, showing: (i) at baseline – the middle arrow shows the point at which the retinal artery and vein exit the optic cup through the lamina cribrosa at its base; (ii) a loss of the inferior NRR at 6 years; and (iii) marked loss of the inferior NRR and subtle loss of the superior NRR at 9 years. Note the position of the blood vessels as they run up over the NRR. c) Cross-sectional view of (i) a normal and (ii) a damaged optic nerve due to glaucoma.

Risk factors and pathophysiology

Of the risk factors identified for glaucoma (see Table 1.2, page 18), age and IOP have the clearest link to pathophysiology.

Age. The prevalence, incidence and progression rate of glaucoma all increase with increasing age, irrespective of IOP. This suggests that older eyes are less able to cope with neurotoxic stress, or that stress factors increase or build up with age. This highlights the importance of the cell biology of the retinal and optic nerve cells in glaucoma.

Intraocular pressure. The prevalence, incidence and progression rate of glaucoma all increase with rising IOP. This suggests that IOP exerts a continuous risk to the retinal ganglion cells in addition to any intrinsic risk. Figure 2.3 shows how the prevalence of glaucoma increases with age and IOP in a compound fashion. For every age group, glaucoma risk increases with higher IOP.

Natural history and prognosis

The natural history of glaucoma is highly variable. If disease onset is late in life and the rate of progression is slow, glaucoma can have relatively

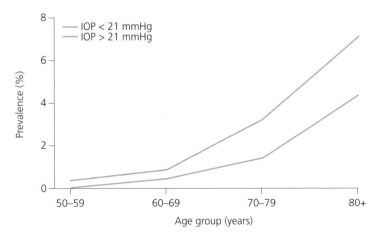

Figure 2.3 The prevalence of open-angle glaucoma according to intraocular pressure (IOP) and age. Source: the Blue Mountains Eye Study. www.cvr.org.au/bmes.htm

minimal impact on activities of daily living. By contrast, when the course of the disease is long or progression is rapid, glaucoma can cause complete and irreversible blindness in both eyes. In general, rate of visual field loss is related to the level of untreated IOP (Table 2.1).

Receptive fields. Optic neurons (ganglion cells) are distributed topographically across the retina and are connected through an intermediary network to the retinal photoreceptors (see Figure 2.1). Many photoreceptors converge on each ganglion cell through the retinal neural network. The area of adjacent photoreceptors that each ganglion cell links to is called its receptive field. To stimulate the receptive field of a ganglion cell, the light falling on it must be sufficiently bright, large and central (Figure 2.4). A more intense light will stimulate ganglion-cell responses in a larger area of the retina. Light falling in the periphery of a receptive field can inhibit rather than stimulate the ganglion cell. Receptive fields vary in size and overlap considerably, particularly in the center of the retina.

The visual field is the total area of the receptive fields, projected into space. The visual fields of the two eyes overlap considerably, facilitating stereovision and making up for any deficiencies in the visual field of each eye (such as the physiological blind spot). This means that losing a small number of ganglion cells may not have a detectable effect on vision, as there are enough remaining cells and

TABLE 2.1

Average time for untreated early-stage disease to progress to end-stage blindness at different intraocular pressures

Pressure (mmHg)	Duration (years)
21–25	14.4
26–30	6.5
> 30	2.9

Adapted from Jay JL, Murdoch JR. The rate of visual field loss in untreated primary open angle glaucoma. *Br J Ophthalmol* 1993;77:176–8.

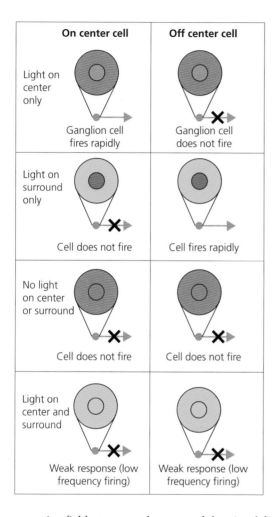

Figure 2.4 The receptive field of a retinal ganglion cell: a region of space in which the presence of a stimulus will alter the firing of the cell.

receptive fields to cover that area of the visual field. Depending on the sensitivity of the visual field test, up to 50% of ganglion cells can be lost before a visual field defect is detectable. Once the visual reserve is exhausted, however, further loss of ganglion cells causes rapid loss of the visual field.

Patterns of visual field loss. It appears that not all of the optic nerve axons are equally susceptible to glaucomatous damage. Neurons at the supero- and inferotemporal regions of the neural rim of the optic disc appear to be most susceptible to damage (see Figure 2.2b ii and iii),

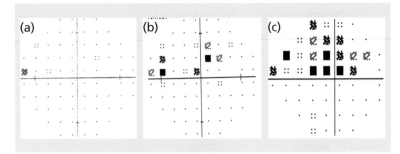

Figure 2.5 The visual field of the eye shown in Figure 3.20 (page 53) over time: (a) at baseline; (b) after 6 years; and (c) after 9 years. A black square is a point in the visual field where light cannot be seen. A black dot is a point where light can be seen. Each square (or dot) is 6 degrees apart. The point where the dark lines cross is the center of vision (fixation). Note how the loss of the upper visual field lies initially on the nasal side and spreads across to fixation.

followed by the temporal rim and lastly the nasal rim. The pattern of visual field loss in glaucoma follows the topographic pattern of axonal damage. In general, glaucoma initially affects the nasal visual field (inferior, superior or both) and spreads centrally to the horizontal midline from the hemifield, reflecting the anatomy of the retinal ganglion cells. If the initial loss is in the periphery of the nasal field, it usually also spreads temporally to the point of fixation at the center of the foveal visual field (Figure 2.5). Visual field loss can progress over a period ranging from weeks to decades. During this time the visual field defect (scotoma) can deepen, widen or both.

What does the patient experience? The effect on the patient depends on where scotomas are located, how dense they are and whether they are unilateral or bilateral. For an adult, a small shallow peripheral scotoma in the upper nasal visual field of one eye might have no effect on daily visual activities. Under careful testing conditions, it might be briefly noticed as an area of vision that is a little duller than the surrounding areas. By contrast, a bilateral scotoma of the same size at fixation (the center of vision) would be very disabling.

The experience of visual field loss is further complicated by a brain process known as 'completion', in which areas of the missing visual field are filled in with information from surrounding areas. As a result, even extensive visual field loss resulting from glaucoma is not usually experienced as black clouds or missing areas of vision.

In addition, it is normal for visual acuity outside the most central visual field to be very poor. Appreciation of detail in a scene comes from multiple rapid fixations to different parts of the scene from the central (foveal) visual field. Thus, everything may look normal to an individual with extensive field loss outside the fovea. Instead, the person may experience objects suddenly jumping into view, apparently from nowhere. When reading, a patient may keep losing their place or perhaps notice a blurring or graying of words just outside their current reading position.

In the later stages of glaucoma, as visual field loss splits the center of vision, the patient's vision darkens, a perception that may initially come and go over hours. Central visual acuity then starts to fall quite rapidly; the ability to read even the largest chart letters will usually be lost within weeks or months. At the end stage of the disease a little temporal visual field may persist with 'hand movements' vision before dropping to perception of light, then no perception of light.

The ultimate stage of glaucoma depends on the length of time the disease remains untreated and the rate of progression. Probably the most important factors in the perception of vision loss are whether the same parts of the visual field of each eye are affected and how close the affected visual field is to fixation (Figure 2.6). Because the visual fields of the eyes overlap, the better eye will maintain a normal-appearing visual field, even if the overlapping area from the other eye is badly damaged. Because central vision (within 10 degrees) is much sharper than peripheral vision, a central scotoma will be more easily noticed and have much greater impact on visually intensive tasks such as reading.

Estimating the rate of progression and future disability is one of the most difficult aspects in the management of glaucoma. Our best attempts incorporate known risk factors for progression to estimate future rate; we can then use rate and state to estimate future disability. Figure 2.7 shows a graph of imaginary glaucoma histories on the basis of state, rate and risk factors. 'State' refers to the stage of the disease, or degree of damage, measured by the percentage of neurons remaining.

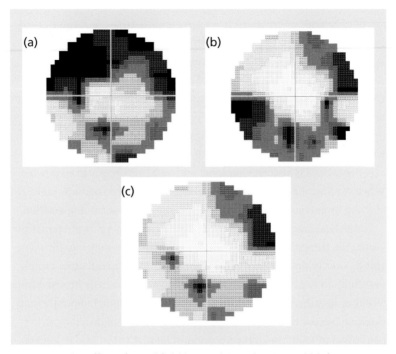

Figure 2.6 The effect of visual field loss on binocular vision: (a) left eye; (b) right eye; (c) both eyes. Because the brain utilizes the best-seeing visual field point, binocular visual loss is best seen when the results of the visual field tests for the two eyes are combined. Here, scotomas in the lower central visual field and upper right field of both eyes cause complete loss of vision in those areas when both eyes are open. The large upper-left scotoma in the left eye (a) has less impact on the vision because of the good vision in the corresponding upper-left field of the right eye (b). Printed courtesy of A. Viswanathan, Moorfields Eye Hospital, London, UK.

The relationship between state and disease impact is not clear cut because of the complicated and bilateral nature of the visual fields (see above). In managing glaucoma, one of our roles is to reduce the slope of the progression line by reducing risk factors.

The rate of glaucoma progression can be measured from the change over a series of visual field tests (usually six tests over 3 years). If none of the risk factors change, future vision loss can be estimated from this rate, a technique that is now used in some visual field analyzer software.

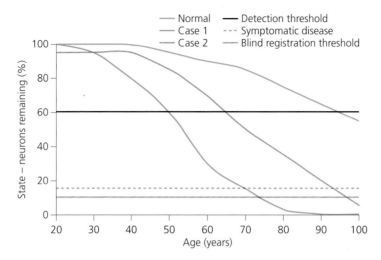

Figure 2.7 The 'state–rate–risk factor' concept of glaucoma. Case 1 has more risk factors for progression than case 2. Arbitrary lines showing the level at which visual field loss may appear in testing and the level that corresponds to blindness are shown. The instantaneous slope of each line represents the rate of neuronal damage at that point in time. The rate of loss is not usually constant over time but depends on changing risk factors, including age. Adapted from Spaeth GL. Visual loss in a glaucoma clinic. I. Sociological considerations. *Invest Ophthalmol* 1970;9:73–82.

Key points – pathophysiology, natural history and prognosis

- In glaucoma, ganglion cells undergo apoptosis from damage at the optic nerve head. This causes a secondary degeneration of neurons of the optic tract.
- Both age and intraocular pressure appear to be continuous risk factors for glaucoma.
- Neurons at the supero- and inferotemporal regions of the neural rim of the optic disc appear to be most susceptible to damage, followed by the temporal rim and lastly the nasal rim.
- Overlap of receptive fields allows up to 50% of ganglion cells to be lost before a visual field defect becomes reproducible.
- Natural history and patient perception are extremely variable.

3 Diagnosis and clinical features

Glaucoma is a chronic optic neuropathy with distinctive structural changes in the optic disc and characteristic functional changes in the visual field (see Chapter 2). Increased intraocular pressure (IOP) is a causal risk factor for glaucoma and is usually the only risk factor that can be treated.

Glaucoma may be primary (of unknown cause) or secondary (of known cause) but findings are quite typical to all types of disease. The diagnosis of all subtypes of glaucoma (see Chapter 1, pages 9–13) requires a relevant history and a detailed eye examination, as described below. The clinical diagnosis of glaucoma is usually based on a combination of IOP measurement, examination of the iridocorneal angle by gonioscopy and examinations of the optic disc and visual field; as such these tests should never be carried out in isolation but should form part of a comprehensive eye examination.

The diagnosis of end-stage glaucoma is straightforward and can be made by any physician trained in the use of the ophthalmoscope. It is, however, preferable to diagnose glaucoma at an early stage, when intervention can alter the course of the disease and change the prognosis.

Diagnosis is far more difficult in the early stages, and has implications of 'labeling' and life-long treatment. The diagnosis is therefore best confirmed by a specialist with expertise not only in slit-lamp examination and measurement of IOP but also in the determination of subtle signs from examination of the optic disc, and proficiency in the interpretation of automated visual fields and imaging techniques.

Box 3.1 provides a useful reminder of the importance of specificity and sensitivity in diagnostic aids.

History
Many patients with primary open-angle glaucoma (OAG) or primary angle-closure glaucoma (ACG) do not volunteer specific symptoms related to the disease. A history of frequent changes of reading glasses may be cause for suspicion, but is not sensitive or specific enough to be

BOX 3.1

A note on the art of diagnosis

The specificity and sensitivity of the history, clinical findings and investigations – in isolation but especially in combination – can be particularly useful to clinicians.

- SpPIN (Specific test, if Positive, rules IN the disease) – a highly specific sign, or test (around 95% specific), if positive, 'rules in' the disease.

- SnNOUT (Sensitive test, if Negative, rules OUT the disease) – a highly sensitive sign or test (around 95% sensitive), if negative, 'rules out' the disease.

More importantly, a combination of results of a lower specificity or sensitivity produces an additive effect to apply these useful clinical rules (see page 55).

Examples

1 Frequency doubling perimetry is a method of assessing the visual field. In the screening mode, the machine usually takes a minute for each eye. Any three abnormal points on the screening mode of the frequency doubling test has a specificity of 99%. Such a finding 'rules in' (confirms) the presence of a field defect.

2 Absence of venous pulsations is 99% sensitive for a diagnosis of papilledema. If venous pulsations are present, the diagnosis can be 'ruled out', at least at that point in time.

used clinically. Patients with advanced disease may present with decreasing visual acuity or a noticeable loss of visual field.

A directed history will help to establish the risk factors for development of the disease and possible causes for the signs of glaucoma. Useful questions to ask the patient when taking a history are summarized in Table 3.1 and are discussed in greater detail below.

Effective communication with the patient at an early stage is important in order to establish a trusting patient–physician relationship. A patient with early-stage glaucoma in particular will rely on the physician to make the correct diagnosis and to initiate appropriate life-long treatment, even though they may not have any specific symptoms.

TABLE 3.1

Questions to ask when taking a detailed history for glaucoma

Medical history

- Do you have, or have you previously had, any of the following systemic conditions?
  - Bronchial asthma
  - Heart block
  - Congestive cardiac failure
  - Migraine
  - Hypertension or hypotension (if so, what is your current treatment?)
  - Diabetes (if so, what is its severity and treatment?)
  - Primary vascular dysregulation (e.g. Raynaud's phenomenon)
  - An episode of profound blood loss (hemorrhage) or hypotension
  - Thyroid eye disease
  - Myasthenia gravis
- Do you have allergies to any medications?

Ocular history

- Have you had to change your reading glasses frequently?
- Have you experienced intermittent blurring of vision?
- Have you experienced episode(s) of pain, redness or watering?
- Have you had any previous diagnosis of raised intraocular pressure or glaucoma?
- Have you received any previous treatment for glaucoma?
- Have you used steroid eye drops for any length of time?
- Have you previously had herpetic eye disease, uveitis or corneal endothelial disease?

CONTINUED

TABLE 3.1 (CONTINUED)

Family history

- Do you have any first-degree relatives (parent or sibling) with glaucoma?
- If so, can you describe the course of the disease in the family and the treatment that was given?
- Has any family member gone blind from glaucoma? If so, at what age?

Social history

- Do you live alone? Can you get assistance with medications (e.g. instilling eye drops) if you need it?
- What/how much alcohol do you drink in a week?
- Do you practice yoga (do you perform head balances or other inverted postures)?
- Do you drink more than half a liter of fluids at a time?

Medical history. Several systemic disorders – e.g. migraine, hypertension, hypotension, primary vascular dysregulation, severe blood loss in the past and thyroid disorders – have been associated with the development of glaucoma (see Table 3.1). Migraine and primary vascular dysregulation probably increase the risk of glaucoma by altering the optic disc perfusion in some way. Profound blood loss in the past can produce findings very similar to glaucoma or can lead to progression of the condition. In addition, comorbid conditions will affect the choice of glaucoma drug treatment; for example, β-blockers can aggravate myasthenia and are contraindicated in patients with asthma or heart block.

Ocular history. The experience of the patient is described in Chapter 2 (see pages 26–7). Although glaucoma is usually asymptomatic, some patients may be able to describe specific ocular symptoms attributed to high IOP. For example, acute angle closure (a less common form of angle closure) may have a dramatic presentation with sudden decrease in vision, pain, redness and watering. Parents of children with congenital glaucoma may have noticed tearing, photophobia, 'large' eyes and a 'hazy' cornea. It is important to take a detailed ocular history because patients may not think to mention that their vision has cleared or that they have had pain if it has receded by the time of the consultation.

Unless specifically asked, patients may not report a past history of steroid usage or even anti-glaucoma eye drops. They may not even report a past history of glaucoma, assuming that treatment resulted in a cure. Others may have forgotten trauma to the eye, an event that can help explain a baffling unilateral glaucoma.

Individuals with myopia are at higher risk for OAG, while those with hypermetropia are at higher risk for ACG.

Family history. A positive family history is an extremely important risk factor for the development of OAG, as it increases the risk of glaucoma up to eightfold; it therefore mandates a careful examination.

It may be helpful to find out more about the treatment close family members (parents and siblings) have undergone, as this may give an indication of the severity of the glaucoma that has been inherited. All first-degree family members of a patient with glaucoma should undergo a comprehensive eye examination. Furthermore, patients must be made aware of hereditary patterns (e.g. of some childhood glaucomas) so they are prepared if they have children of their own. A major problem is that most people do not know whether they have a family history of glaucoma. For some people, what was thought to be a positive family history of glaucoma may be a family history of high IOP without glaucoma (ocular hypertension).

Social history. Does the patient live alone? If medical treatment is being prescribed, it is important to know that the patient can instill eye drops.

Consumption of large quantities of water at a time (as is sometimes prescribed in alternative lifestyles) can be dangerous for patients with glaucoma, as can consumption of large quantities of beer in a short period.

Performing head balances and other inverted postures in yoga increases IOP and could also add to the risk of progression.

Eye examination

To detect glaucoma early and therefore prevent blindness, all individuals who present to an eyecare professional – an ophthalmologist or an optometrist – should undergo a comprehensive eye examination, with visual field testing if the disc findings are suspicious. This will detect not only glaucoma but also most potentially blinding ocular conditions. The main elements of a comprehensive eye examination are described below (Table 3.2).

Table 3.3 shows the findings that increase the likelihood of a glaucoma diagnosis. A diagnosis may not always be possible during the course of one visit: in suspect cases and patients with very early disease it may be necessary to repeat the full examination after a period of observation. In children, some parts of the examination may need to be performed under sedation or anesthesia.

TABLE 3.2

Key elements of a comprehensive eye examination for glaucoma

- Check vision and refraction
- Examine external appearance of the eye
- Assess ocular motility
- Slit-lamp examination
- Examine the pupil, with special attention to the presence of a relative afferent pupillary defect (RAPD; see Figure 3.2)
- Measure intraocular pressure using applanation tonometry
- Examine the angle of the eye by gonioscopy
- Dilate to examine the optic disc and retina (see text)
- Check for functional defects of the visual fields by automated perimetry IF optic disc examination suggests glaucoma

Note: Imaging of the optic disc, nerve fiber layer and angle can be undertaken to confirm diagnosis or to help detect change at follow-up.

TABLE 3.3

Risk factors that suggest a higher probability of glaucoma in a person with an optic disc appearance suspicious for glaucoma

- Increasing age (70 years and over)
- Family history of the disease
- Myopia
- Use of steroids (topical or systemic)
- Raised intraocular pressure (> 22 mmHg)
- Occludable anterior chamber angles on gonioscopy (see text)
- Signs of anterior chamber inflammation, pigment dispersion or pseudoexfoliation

Visual acuity and refraction tests. Visual acuity is conventionally measured one eye at a time using a standard high-contrast Snellen's chart, usually at a distance of 6 meters (20 feet). This is carried out with and without the patient's existing spectacle correction. Improvement of vision with the use of a pinhole suggests a refractive error rather than more sinister pathology.

Refraction performed with streak retinoscopy (or an autorefractometer) followed by subjective refraction determines and corrects any refractive error.

Initial external examination of the eye using a flashlight is important to detect signs of, for example, a subtle hemangioma or dilated episcleral veins, which would suggest a secondary cause of glaucoma. Ciliary congestion suggests sinister intraocular pathology, including acute angle closure.

Ocular motility is assessed using various cover tests, both at a distance and close to the patient, as well as ocular movements in the cardinal positions. Assessment of ocular motility is important because detection of amblyopia or sensory exotropia may affect the management plan. For example, an eye with sensory exotropia and dense amblyopia will not be treated as aggressively as a normal eye with good visual potential.

Slit-lamp examination (before and after pupil dilatation) provides a highly magnified three-dimensional view of the eye surface, anterior chamber, lens, vitreous, retina and optic disc. Any signs of pseudoexfoliation, pigment dispersion, uveitis or trauma can be detected using a slit-lamp microscope.

Pseudoexfoliation is a common cause of glaucoma. Pigment liberation following dilatation is highly suggestive of pseudoexfoliation; any indication of pigment liberation should direct the search for subtle signs of glaucoma such as the early 'brown' stage in which brown pigment may be seen in a radial disposition on the periphery of the lens following dilatation (Figure 3.1).

Corneal edema. Hydration of the cornea decreases its resistance to flattening. Thus, corneal edema detected during such an examination may mean that the IOP measurement has been underestimated.

Posterior synechiae may explain distortion of the pupil and direct suspicion towards a diagnosis of uveitis or other causes of such a finding rather than glaucoma.

Examination of the pupil. Glaucoma is usually an asymmetric disease. Demonstration of a relative afferent pupillary defect (RAPD; an abnormal response in which one pupil dilates, rather than constricts, when a light is shone alternately on it and the other eye) is an important diagnostic clue (Figure 3.2) – as an RAPD occurs only in the face of major asymmetric loss of nerve fibers, it may be a prognostic factor as well. A pupil dilated from iris muscle damage can be a sign of acute angle closure.

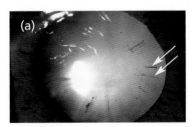 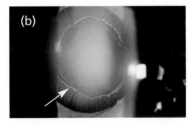

Figure 3.1 (a) The early 'brown' stage of pseudoexfoliation, characterized by radial streaks of pigment on the periphery of the lens. (b) Classic pseudoexfoliation syndrome, showing deposition of pigment on the lens.

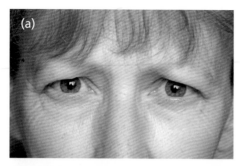

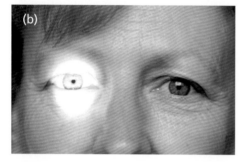

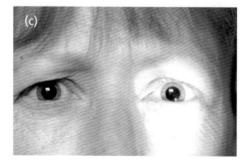

Figure 3.2 Testing for a relative afferent pupillary defect (RAPD) using the swinging light test: (a) normal size of pupils with room lights on; (b) room lights are turned down, the patient looks into the distance and a light is shone onto the right eye – the patient shows a normal response with constriction of both pupils; (c) dilation of both pupils after suddenly swinging the light to the left eye, indicating a left RAPD. Source: *Fast Facts: Ophthalmology*.

Measurement of intraocular pressure. The gold standard for measuring IOP is the Goldmann applanation tonometer attached to the slit-lamp microscope (Figure 3.3); handheld instruments such as the Perkins tonometer or the electronic tonopen may also be used. Applanation tonometry is a contact method for measuring IOP. Local anesthetic eye drops are administered and fluorescein instilled. The tonometer enables the physician to determine the force required to flatten a defined part of the cornea. Since this force depends on the IOP, the tonometer can be calibrated so that the pressure is read from a graduated dial.

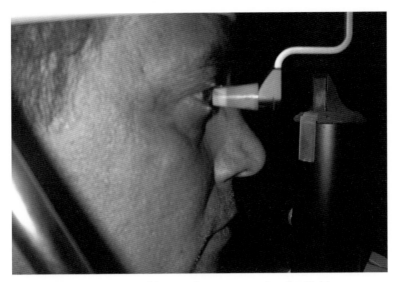

Figure 3.3 Measurement of intraocular pressure using the Goldmann applanation tonometer attached to a slit-lamp microscope.

The Goldmann applanation tonometer, like any other method of measurement, may be subject to errors; measurements must be performed carefully to avoid erroneous readings. For example, corneal thickness affects IOP (see Corneal edema, page 37), so this must be taken into account during measurement.

A non-contact (air-puff) tonometer may be a useful way to check the IOP in busy clinics. All abnormal values (after repetition) should be rechecked by the applanation method. The role of newer tonometers such as the Pascal and Ocular Response Analyzer are being investigated. IOP in all patients with glaucoma should be measured using applanation tonometry (Goldmann or Perkins).

Interpretation of IOP readings. Glaucoma becomes more likely as IOP increases. While the risk increases throughout the IOP range, a sensible cut-off to define a 'high' IOP is two standard deviations above the population mean. The two standard deviations value varies between populations, but a value greater than 21 mmHg is a reasonable cut-off for most Caucasian and Asian populations. The mean IOP and cut-off level are lower for Japanese and Korean populations (18 mmHg).

A 'high' IOP is reasonably specific (although 'SpPin' is not applicable, as it does not achieve the required 95% specificity; see Box 3.1, page 31) but is not sensitive for glaucoma. Accordingly, a high IOP may suggest glaucoma but a reading in the normal range does not rule it out. Glaucoma is much more likely when an eye with a high IOP has evidence of damage to the trabecular meshwork (e.g. angle closure or trauma).

Multiple readings. As with any measurement, a single raised reading cannot be relied upon, particularly in the absence of other signs of disease. Even if other signs of the disease are present, measurements should be repeated, not just to detect raised IOP but also to obtain a baseline to enable evaluation of the effects of treatment.

Diurnal fluctuation in IOP. IOP normally fluctuates by up to 5 mmHg over the course of the day; this may be more in glaucoma. If IOP appears 'normal' or 'low' in a patient with damage to the optic disc or visual field, multiple readings obtained at different times of the day (and even night) may be desirable. This should certainly be considered before initiating any expensive or invasive investigations to look for non-glaucomatous damage. The principle of multiple readings, preferably obtained at different times of the day, applies even after treatment is initiated. The IOP should be measured at every visit.

Assessment of the iridocorneal angle. Total internal reflection in the cornea makes it impossible to view the iridocorneal angle structures directly, even with the slit-lamp microscope. A special contact lens is needed to overcome this phenomenon. Gonioscopy using such a lens is used to examine the iridocorneal angle of the eye's anterior chamber (Figure 3.4). It is best performed using an 'indentation' type of gonioscope. The distance between the trabecular meshwork and iris (angle), the thickness and curvature of the peripheral iris and the state of the trabecular meshwork are important factors in angle assessment. A normal angle seen by gonioscopy is shown in Figure 3.5.

Gonioscopy is not a one-time event. A patient with OAG and narrow angles can develop angle closure over time, so gonioscopy must be repeated at least annually if the signs of the disease change, and also after interventions like iridotomy, trabeculectomy or cataract removal (see Chapter 6).

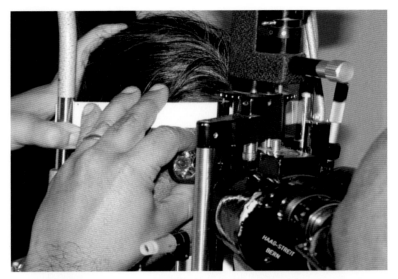

Figure 3.4 Gonioscopy: a special mirrored contact lens is used to measure the angle of the anterior chamber.

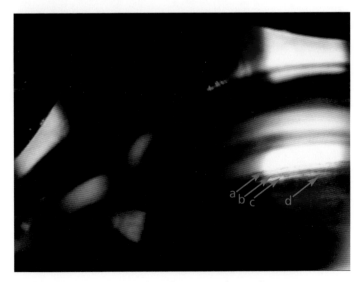

Figure 3.5 Normal iridocorneal angle, as seen by gonioscopy:
(a) Schwalbe's line; (b) trabecular meshwork; (c) scleral spur;
(d) ciliary body band.

Optimum testing conditions. The testing conditions are critical in determining if an angle is open or closed. Most angles will 'open' if the examination is performed in a bright room with a long slit beam that impinges on and constricts the pupil, and/or pressure is applied by the gonioscope (Figure 3.6). The ideal testing conditions therefore comprise:

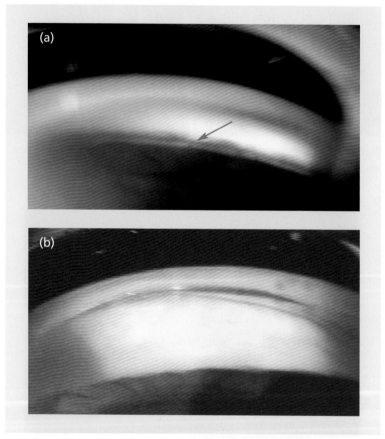

Figure 3.6 Change in angle with change in illumination. (a) Gonioscopy performed in bright illumination constricts the pupil and reveals the angle structures (arrowed), leading to a wrong diagnosis of open angle.
(b) When optimum conditions are used (see text), the trabecular meshwork is no longer visible and the correct diagnosis of angle closure can be made.

- dim room illumination
- low-intensity slit-lamp illumination
- a low slit-beam height (so that light does not impinge on the pupil)
- no pressure on the eye from the gonioscope.

The operator should wait 30–45 seconds for the pupil to dilate before deciding if the angle is open. If the posterior trabecular meshwork is not visible under these conditions, the patient should be asked to look towards the mirror in order to obtain an 'over the (iris) hill' view of the angle (Figure 3.7). If more than 180 degrees of the posterior trabecular meshwork is visible in this 'over-the-hill' view, the angle can be considered open.

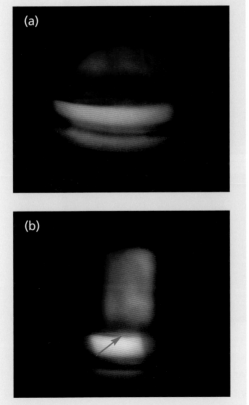

Figure 3.7 (a) In relative pupillary block increased pressure in the posterior chamber causes a bulge ('hill') in the mid-peripheral iris; when the patient looks straight ahead, this 'hill' can obstruct the view of an otherwise open angle. No angle structures are visible and the angle is labeled as closed. (b) The patient is asked to look towards the direction of the mirror. The mirror is now ideally positioned for an 'over the hill' view into the angle. As the trabecular meshwork is now visible (arrowed), the angle is actually 'open'.

Indentation gonioscopy. Once the nature of the angle has been established, the intensity of illumination and slit-beam height can be raised to constrict the pupil, and 'indentation' gonioscopy can be performed to look for other signs of pathology in the angle. Pressure is applied with the gonioscope lens against the surface of the eye, pushing the cornea backwards and increasing the IOP within the anterior chamber. The fluid is not compressible, so the lens and iris are also pushed backwards, opening the iridocorneal angle. This enables the operator to look for the peripheral anterior synechiae (Figure 3.8), consequences of angle closure or inflammation, and signs of pseudoexfoliation, trauma, old hemorrhage, inflammation or new vessels.

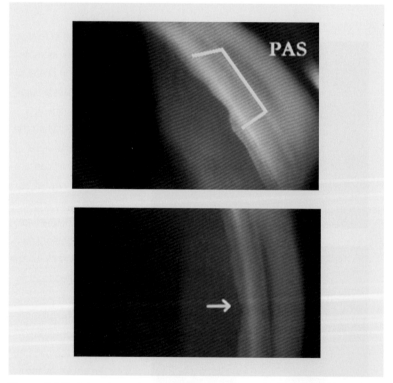

Figure 3.8 Peripheral anterior synechiae. Note how the iris is pulled over the trabecular meshwork, obstructing aqueous flow. Reproduced courtesy of Dr Kalyani Prasad, consultant ophthalmologist in private practice, Hyderabad, India.

Imaging techniques. The ultrasound biomicrosope (UBM) provides high-resolution images of the angle structures and the ciliary body (Figure 3.9). It is a useful tool to assess the anterior segment, including the angle, when a hazy or opaque cornea precludes visualization. It is also useful in diagnosing conditions that affect the ciliary body, including pathology associated with glaucoma. Older UBMs require a water bath and a trained technician and are therefore not practical for routine clinical use. Newer UBMs do not require a water bath and may be more useful clinically.

Anterior segment optical coherence tomography (AS-OCT) can also be used to visualize the anterior segment and angle of the eye (Figure 3.10). AS-OCT is particularly good at showing changes with

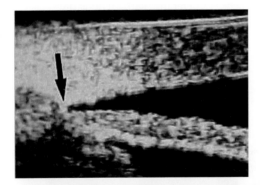

Figure 3.9 Cross-section of the angle of the anterior chamber obtained by ultrasound biomicroscopy. The arrow shows the location of the scleral spur.

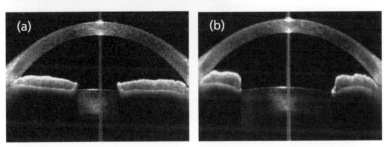

Figure 3.10 The effect of ambient illumination on angle configuration shown with AS-OCT imaging. (a) In the light, the pupil constricts, rendering the iris profile regular and widening the angle recess. (b) In the dark, the pupil dilates, increasing pupil block and appositionally closing the angle. Reproduced with permission from Covar RA, Healey PR. Occludable angles. In: *Angle Closure Glaucoma*. Eds C Hong, T Yamamoto. Amsterdam: Kugler, 2007.

illumination. Unlike UBM, it does not resolve detail behind the iris.

Examination of the optic disc and retina. Indirect ophthalmoscopy will provide a low-magnification overall view of the posterior pole of the retina, and is an essential procedure for examination of the periphery of the retina. However, because of its low magnification, the indirect ophthalmoscope is not suitable for examination of the optic disc. While a direct ophthalmoscope in experienced hands is useful, a magnified stereoscopic examination of the optic disc, using a 60–90 D lens or a contact lens with the slit-lamp microscope, is required (Figure 3.11).

Findings should be documented, preferably with an optic disc photograph but at least a drawing for comparison with future

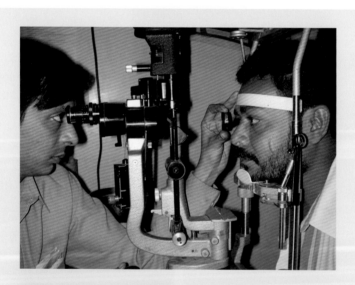

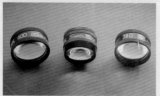

Figure 3.11 Fundus examination using the slit-lamp microscope and special lenses.

examinations. Stereophotographs are the gold standard and allow careful review, as well as documentation to detect changes on follow-up. Structural defects in the optic disc in glaucoma are numerous. As diagnosis is based on a combination of signs, a systematic approach to disc assessment is required (Table 3.4).

Increased cup-to-disc ratio (CDR). Most people have about 1 million axons that exit the eye through the disc, forming the neuroretinal rim (NRR; described in more detail below), irrespective of the size of the optic disc. The optic cup can be thought of as the 'space' that is left over after these axons have been accommodated in the disc. The size of the optic disc varies considerably and the space left over (i.e. the cup) has to vary according to the size of the disc. Accordingly, a small disc may not have any cup, while a large disc may have a large cup.

In glaucoma, the optic cup enlarges as nerve tissue is destroyed. A large CDR is a common sign of glaucomatous damage. In general, a CDR above 0.7 suggests a higher likelihood of glaucoma. However, as Figure 3.12 shows, the distribution of CDR varies widely within a population; therefore, CDR should not be used in isolation. For

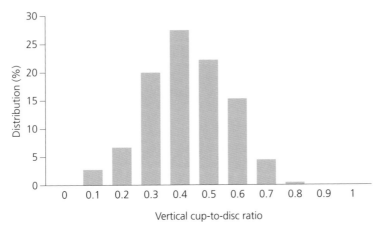

Figure 3.12 Distribution of vertical cup-to-disc ratios in participants in the Blue Mountains Eye Study. Reproduced with permission from Mitchell P, Smith W, Attebo K, Healey PR. Prevalence of open-angle glaucoma in Australia: the Blue Mountains Eye Study. *Ophthalmology* 1996;103:1661–9.

TABLE 3.4

Systematic approach to optic disc assessment

- Assess optic disc size and shape
  - The edge of the disc is the inner edge of the thin white ring that surrounds most optic discs: small discs ≤ 1.3 mm should have small cups; large discs > 2.0 mm may have large cups
  - Most discs are slightly vertically oval or round
  - Abnormally shaped discs may have an abnormal neuroretinal rim in the absence of disease
  - Tilted discs often have notches
  - Extremely large discs often have very large cup-to-disc ratios (CDRs)
- Observe the neuroretinal rim
  - 'ISNT' rule should apply: Inferior > Superior > Nasal > Temporal (see Figure 3.17, page 51) is the pattern of thickness in 85% of normal discs
  - Presence of a notch is suggestive of glaucoma if the disc shape is normal. A notch to the optic disc margin is very suggestive of glaucoma
  - Calculate the vertical CDR by expressing the sum of the thinnest superior and inferior neural rim widths as a fraction of the largest vertical disc diameter (CDR > 0.7 suggests glaucoma)
- Look for optic disc hemorrhages
  - Optic disc hemorrhages are suggestive of glaucoma and confer a high (30%) 10-year risk of developing glaucoma in an otherwise normal eye
- Observe the parapapillary region
  - Beta zone parapapillary atrophy is seen in about 1 in 5 normal discs but also in areas adjacent to rim notching or disc hemorrhage
- Examine the nerve fiber layer (NFL)
  - Diffuse NFL loss appears as a general reduction in brightness
  - Localized NFL loss appears as wedge-shaped dark areas emanating from the optic disc
- Observe the lamina cribrosa for an acquired pit of the optic nerve (rare)

example, a CDR of 0.5 may be abnormal for a small disc, while a CDR of 0.7 may be normal for a very large disc. Consequently, the CDR may be useful but only if it is related to the size of the disc (Figure 3.13).

Disc size can be easily estimated on the slit-lamp microscope with a 60 D lens. A narrow slit-beam height is adjusted vertically until it just encompasses the margins of the optic disc (Figure 3.14). Generally, a disc with a vertical diameter ≤ 1.3 mm is considered small, 1.4–2 mm is considered medium and > 2 mm is considered large. People of European

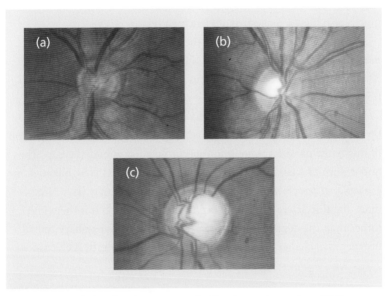

Figure 3.13 Relationship between optic disc size and cupping. All three images show normal discs, illustrating that the size of the cup depends on the size of the disc: (a) is a small disc and hence has no cup; (b) is a medium-sized disc with cupping; (c) is a large disc with a large cup.

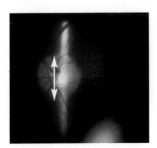

Figure 3.14 Measurement of disc size with a slit-lamp microscope.

extraction generally have smaller discs (mean 1.5 mm) whereas African and Indian people have larger discs (mean 1.8 mm). It is not important to obtain an actual measurement but to know whether a disc is small, medium or large. As with any other clinical measurement, this only becomes possible after examining and measuring a large number of discs.

Cup size. The question to ask is: 'Should this disc normally have this sort of cup?' A small CDR (e.g. 0.3) is usually considered to be in the normal range but may be abnormal in a small disc; on the other hand, a large cup may by normal in a large disc. An increase in the cup over time is also highly suggestive of glaucoma (Figure 3.15).

Cup-to-disc ratio asymmetry. If the CDR in the two eyes differs by more than 0.2 after accounting for differences in the size of the two discs, the possibility of glaucomatous damage should be considered (Figure 3.16).

Neuroretinal rim. This is the area of the optic disc that is occupied by the axons and requires a thorough investigation. Direct examination of this tissue provides more information than examining the cup. The importance of examining the neuroretinal rim (NRR) is highlighted, for example, in people with myopia. Although myopes may have large discs, the thin sclera limits the 'depth' of cupping and it is the width rather than the depth that is important. Myopic parapapillary retinal degenerative changes also make examination difficult. In such cases of

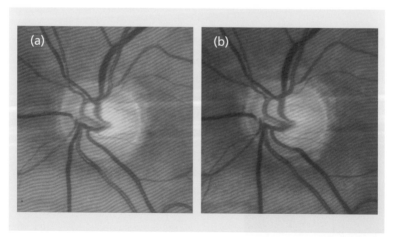

Figure 3.15 Increase in cup size over time.

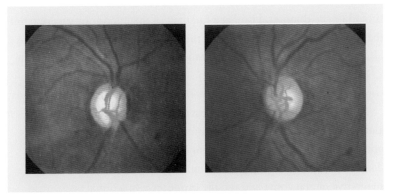

Figure 3.16 Cup-to-disc ratio asymmetry between the two eyes.

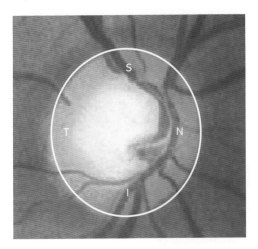

Figure 3.17 'ISNT' rule: the inferior area of the rim is usually the thickest, followed by the superior area, the nasal area and then the temporal area.

doubt, the use of a contact lens (a two- or three-mirror Goldmann lens) provides a good stereoscopic view of the NRR. Defects in the NRR suggest pathology, as described below.

Pattern of thickness. The NRR of a healthy optic disc varies by sector: the inferior area of the rim is usually the thickest, followed by the superior area, the nasal area and then the temporal area (Figure 3.17); this is known as the 'ISNT' rule. There may be normal variations, but change in this pattern suggests glaucomatous pathology; for example, if the inferior area of the rim is thinner than the superior, that could suggest pathology. Certainly, an inferior or superior rim that is equal to or thinner than the temporal rim is highly suspect, as the temporal rim should be the thinnest. Localized thinning of the inferior or superior rim that does not extend to the edge of the disc (peripapillary scleral rim) is also suspect. **Assessment of the rim-to-disc ratio is more useful than the CDR.** A rim-to-disc ratio of less than 0.1:1 in any area should be considered pathological.

Neuroretinal rim notch. Focal loss of rim tissue is common in glaucoma. A localized area of loss of the neuroretinal rim is called a notch. A notch can be within the rim tissue or can extend to the optic disc margin (peripapillary scleral ring) (Figure 3.18). A notch is highly suggestive of glaucoma and usually produces a functional visual field defect.

Optic disc hemorrhage. A retinal hemorrhage that touches the NRR is relatively rare in normal eyes but is strongly associated with glaucoma and its future development (Figure 3.19).

Parapapillary chorioretinal atrophy (beta zone) is quite common, found in about 20% of the older population. It is more common in people with myopia and glaucoma. In an eye with glaucoma it is often found adjacent to rim loss, and increases in size as the glaucoma progresses (Figure 3.20).

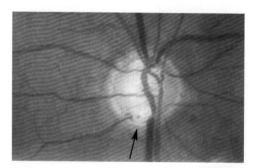

Figure 3.18 Neuroretinal rim notch (arrowed).

Figure 3.19 Optic disc hemorrhage, touching the neuroretinal rim.

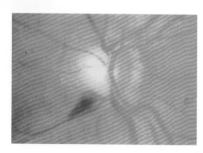

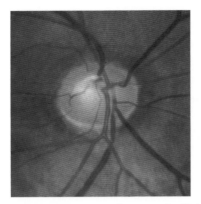 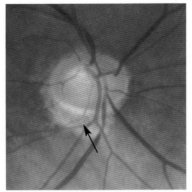

Figure 3.20 Parapapillary atrophy (lighter area around black arrowhead) developing with open-angle glaucoma over 9 years. The visual field of this patient is shown in Figure 2.5 (page 26).

Acquired pit of the optic nerve. An acquired pit is a discrete oval-shaped depression in the lamina cribrosa (Figure 3.21). It is usually associated with localized excavation of the neuroretinal rim. The presence of an acquired pit of the optic nerve (APON) is strongly associated with glaucoma. It is usually located in the inferotemporal or superotemporal sectors of the disc. A congenital pit of the optic nerve is rarer and is not associated with glaucoma.

Nerve fiber layer (NFL) defect. The NFL should be examined on well-focused and illuminated optic disc photographs or using a green filter on the slit-lamp microscope or ophthalmoscope. The green light is reflected by the NFL and is absorbed by the pigment in the retinal

Figure 3.21 Acquired pit of the optic nerve (arrowed). Reproduced with permission from Healey PR, Mitchell P. The prevalence of optic disc pits and their relationship to glaucoma. *J Glaucoma* 2008;17:11–14.

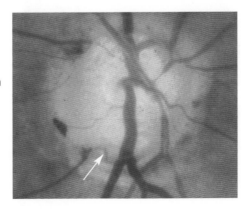

epithelium and choroid layers to create a dark background. The normal arcuate NFL appears as fine bright striations. Viewed from the superior arcuate NFL to the inferior NFL, a bright–dark–bright pattern is visible, the dark area being the region between the disc and the macula (Figure 3.22). The inferior arcuate NFL is a larger area and is easier to see than the superior arcuate NFL.

A localized NFL defect appears as a dark wedge that follows the pattern of the NFL (Figure 3.23). Characteristically a defect:

- is wider than an arteriole
- touches the edge of the disc
- increases in width towards the periphery.

Such defects have a strong predictive value for future functional changes. The specificity is very high ('SpPIN'; see Box 3.1, page 31) but the sensitivity is poor. The defects are a definite sign of pathology, but can also occur in diseases other than glaucoma. Localized defects are sometimes easily seen on indirect ophthalmoscopy.

Diffuse NFL defects are more difficult to detect because the normal bright–dark–bright pattern is lost. The pattern looks more like dark–dark–dark (Figure 3.24). Better visibility of the superior NFL defect relative to the inferior NFL is also suspect.

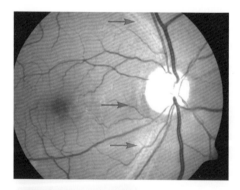

Figure 3.22 Normal retinal nerve fiber layer, showing distinct bright–dark–bright striations (arrowed).

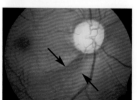

Figure 3.23 Localized (wedge-shaped) retinal nerve fiber layer defect, increasing in width towards the periphery.

Figure 3.24 Diffuse retinal nerve fiber layer defect with a dark–dark–dark pattern. Reproduced courtesy of Professor Jost Jonas, University of Mannheim, Germany.

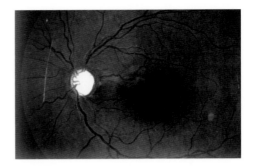

NFL defects are often more clearly visible on well-focused well-exposed color photographs than by direct clinical observation because even bright illumination of the NFL makes darker areas more visible.

Pseudo-NFL defects are most commonly seen where the main superior and inferior nerve fiber bundles are split. NFL defects are also found in eyes with non-glaucomatous optic neuropathies and occasionally in otherwise normal eyes.

Diagnosis from optic disc examination

The diagnosis of glaucoma can be made quite easily when comparing two photographs of the same optic disc taken 10 years apart (see Figure 2.2, page 22). However, because of the enormous variation in the appearance of a normal optic disc, it can be difficult to decide whether a disc has suffered glaucomatous damage on the basis of just one examination. As some of the signs of glaucoma can be seen in a normal disc, glaucomatous damage to the optic nerve is usually assumed from a combination of signs (Table 3.5).

For example, in a disc with a notch as well as an NFL defect, the combined specificity is high enough to 'rule in' glaucoma. Similarly, in a disc with thinning of the rim as well as an optic disc hemorrhage, the specificity is high enough to 'rule in' glaucoma. On the other hand, the sensitivity of individual signs is not high enough to 'rule out' glaucoma unless most, or all, the signs are absent.

Where there is only one sign, it is particularly important that disc appearance corresponds with the visual field result.

TABLE 3.5

Syndromic diagnosis of glaucoma

In a normally shaped optic disc, two or more of the following signs, or one of the following signs plus a matching visual field loss, indicates glaucoma:

- Neuronal retinal rim notch (note: a tilted optic disc can have an abnormal neural rim without having glaucoma)
- Vertical cup-to-disc ratio > 0.7, or rim-to-disc ratio ≤ 0.1 at any one point outside the temporal area
- Optic disc hemorrhage
- Focal or diffuse nerve fiber layer loss
- Acquired pit of the optic nerve

The simplest rule to help with the diagnosis of glaucomatous damage at the optic disc is thus: unless proved otherwise, *all* optic discs have glaucomatous changes. This rule emphasizes that in order to detect glaucoma we must have a high index of suspicion and examine all patients carefully.

In individuals with established glaucoma the optic disc should be examined at every visit, in particular to look for optic disc hemorrhages, which can come and go over a few weeks. Depending on the course of the disease, documentation should be updated every 6–12 months (see Chapter 7).

Imaging the optic disc

Imaging techniques for the optic nerve and/or NFL include Heidelberg retinal tomography, optical coherence tomography and NFL analysis (see Chapter 7). The World Glaucoma Association consensus on imaging states that these instruments lack the sensitivity and specificity for routine clinical use. In the hands of experts, however, they may provide valuable clinical information. We believe that imaging devices may have a major role to play in the important area of documenting and detecting change.

Visual field

Glaucoma is a potentially blinding disease because it causes visual field defects that can affect visual function. Once such a defect is detected, diagnosis and management decisions become clearer. The detection of visual field defects and their progression (or stability) is therefore extremely important in the management of glaucoma. As with any other test, the visual field should be assessed *only* if disease is suspected; a field 'defect' in a person whose disc examination is normal is likely to be a false positive.

Assessment of visual field by any method has a strong subjective element. Automated perimetry, the gold standard for assessment of visual field, makes the test as objective as possible. Calibrated perimeters that have been previously validated must be used. Automated perimetry is associated with a learning curve (see pages 60–1), so it is best not to rely on the first two or three fields.

The perimetry printout can be analyzed systematically in zones (Figure 3.25). The field defects in glaucoma are usually localized, and these localized defects will show up in both the total-deviation and pattern-deviation plots (Figure 3.26a). A generalized depression is more characteristic of anterior segment-related causes such as cataract affecting the visual field; generalized defects are limited to the total-deviation plot (Figure 3.26b).

The results of visual field tests must never be interpreted in isolation. The field should correlate with structural damage to the optic disc and NFL (Figure 3.27). In early glaucoma, structural damage can be apparent before detectable field loss. Similarly, but more rarely, glaucomatous field loss can be found in the absence of detectable disc damage. Such a lack of correlation substantially weakens the certainty of diagnosis and warrants careful re-evaluation using varied methods of assessment. For example, a patient with glaucomatous disc damage but no associated field loss seen on standard automated perimetry may show field loss when short wavelength or frequency doubling perimetry is performed (and vice versa). A glaucomatous field defect in the presence of an apparently normal optic disc may have a number of causes, but detection of a matching focal NFL defect photographically in the presence of raised IOP would add certainty to a diagnosis of glaucoma.

57

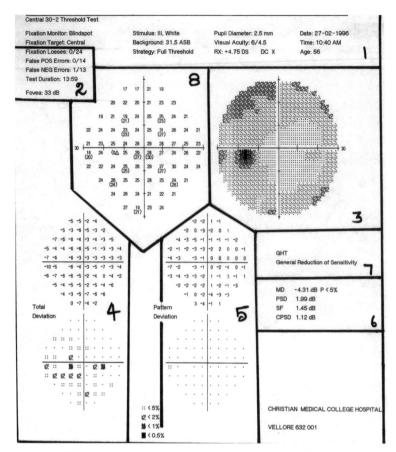

Figure 3.25 Perimetry printout of a normal visual field, split into zones for analysis. Zone 1: patient and test information. Zone 2: reliability indices and foveal threshold. Zone 3: gray scale (not relied on to make a diagnosis). Zone 4: total-deviation plot, showing a point-by-point comparison of the patient's visual sensitivity with age-related normal values, which calls attention to any generalized sinking of the hill of vision but cannot confirm the presence of a diagnostic localized scotoma. Zone 5: pattern-deviation plot, showing the deviation of the individual points from age-related normal values after adjusting for any generalized depression of the hill of vision. To confirm a localized scotoma, the dark spots on the total-deviation plot must persist in the pattern-deviation plot. Zone 6: global indices. Zone 7: glaucoma hemifield test. Zone 8: actual visual threshold values at the tested points.

(a)

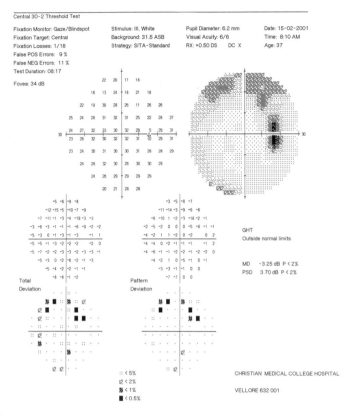

(b)

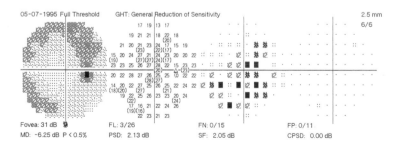

Figure 3.26 Perimetry printouts of: (a) a localized early glaucomatous visual field defect; (b) a generalized cataract field defect.

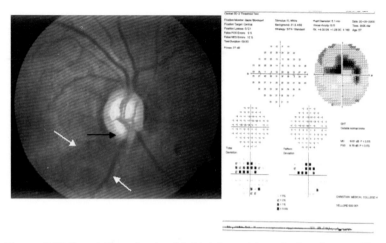

Figure 3.27 Correlation of a visual field defect with optic disc changes. The optic disc shows thinning of the inferior rim (black arrow) and a wedge-shaped defect of the nerve fiber layer inferiorly (white arrows). This correlates with the visual field defect: a scotoma primarily in the superior part of the total-deviation plot that persists on the pattern-deviation plot. Note the arcuate-shaped defect on the gray scale. The gray scale should never be used for interpretation but is useful to demonstrate the defect to the patient.

Follow-up. Once the diagnosis of glaucoma is confirmed, management decisions are based on the detection of progression seen in repeated examinations of the optic disc and serial visual field tests (see Chapter 7). It is important to have a baseline assessment of the visual field for comparison. Baseline visual fields are best obtained early in the course of the disease and should not include fields obtained during the learning curve. The learning curve varies from individual to individual; most patients usually require two or three fields to get over this curve (Figure 3.28). Two fields obtained after the learning curve constitute the baseline against which subsequent fields can be compared in order to detect disease progression.

Progression is generally detected using the Glaucoma Progression Analysis (GPA) and the Visual Field Index Summary (VFI), both of which are discussed in Chapter 7. The decision as to whether a visual field defect is progressing is made by correlating the clinical course

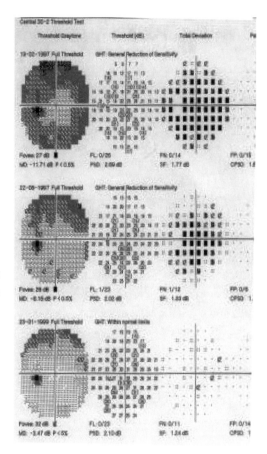

Figure 3.28 The visual field test is associated with a learning curve. The decrease in black spots on the total-deviation plot over time illustrates the effect of the learning curve. For this reason, the first two or three fields should be ignored.

(disc changes, IOP, lack of other findings to explain the field) with the Overview and GPA printouts.

When to suspect glaucoma

After taking a thorough history and conducting a comprehensive eye examination, glaucoma should be suspected when one or more of the signs in Table 3.5 (see page 56) are found. In addition, the possibility of glaucoma should be entertained in all individuals with IOP > 21 mmHg (ocular hypertensive), or with a trabecular meshwork that is visible on gonioscopy for less than 180 degrees (primary angle closure suspects; see below), on the basis that the prevalence and risk of glaucoma is higher in these groups.

61

Clinical features of glaucoma subtypes

Primary open-angle glaucoma (OAG) is a chronic, slowly progressive, bilateral but frequently asymmetric disease. OAG occurs in adults with an 'open' and normal appearing anterior chamber angle on gonioscopy with no other cause for the findings. IOP is a causal risk factor, and at present is the only one that can be manipulated for therapeutic benefit.

The diagnosis of primary OAG is one of exclusion. The angle must be 'open' on gonioscopy and there should be no signs of secondary glaucoma.

Differential diagnosis. The demonstration of an open angle is particularly important in regions of the world where primary ACG is common and needs to be ruled out. Primary OAG can occur without raised IOP, and primary ACG can imitate primary OAG in individuals with a normal IOP. Before initiating expensive or invasive investigations, multiple IOP readings should be taken to rule out raised IOP, and clinical examination (including gonioscopy) should be repeated. A single peripheral anterior synechiae in an individual suspected of having primary ACG can make the diagnosis.

An optic disc that is damaged as a result of neurological causes shows pallor disproportionate to and beyond the area of cupping. The changes in the NRR characteristic of glaucoma are not usually seen. The ISNT pattern of the rim (see Figure 3.17, page 51) is usually preserved.

Primary angle closure disease (PACD). The spectrum of PACD includes:
- primary angle-closure suspects (PACS)
- primary angle closure (PAC)
- primary ACG.

While the majority of patients with PACD, including primary ACG, are asymptomatic, angle closure can present with acute symptoms of decreased vision associated with raised IOP (usually above 30 mmHg), pain, redness and watering. In this condition, referred to as acute angle closure (AAC), the high IOP can damage the optic disc via the mechanism of glaucoma (AACG) or by an acute and probably ischemic effect. This second form of optic nerve damage is characterized by pallor rather than cupping of the NRR. Both mechanisms and therefore signs can be present together.

Primary angle-closure suspects is the term used to describe patients without glaucoma whose angles are at risk of closure but who have no structural or functional signs of trabecular meshwork damage (also known as occludable angles or anatomically narrow angles). On gonioscopy, the posterior trabecular meshwork is visible for less than 180 degrees. On indentation gonioscopy there are no peripheral anterior synechiae or signs of angle closure.

Primary angle closure. As in PACS, the posterior trabecular meshwork is visible for less than 180 degrees. In addition, the IOP is raised and/or there are peripheral anterior synechiae in the angle.

Primary angle-closure glaucoma. In addition to the signs of PAC, these patients have glaucomatous damage to the optic disc and, when the damage is sufficient, defects in the visual field.

Differential diagnosis. Changes in IOP, the optic disc and the visual field are common to both primary OAG and primary ACG, so they must be differentiated on the basis of gonioscopy. It cannot be overemphasized that the treatment of PAC and primary ACG is diametrically opposite to that of primary OAG. PAC and early primary ACG can potentially be cured by laser iridotomy, thereby preventing progression to blindness. The distinction between primary OAG and PACD is therefore crucial.

Differential diagnoses of AAC are listed in Table 3.6. Congestion limited to the region around the limbus (ciliary congestion) suggests a more serious cause. Raised IOP and dilated pupils distinguish AAC from acute uveitis. New vessels on the iris coupled with raised IOP provides a diagnosis of secondary (neovascular) glaucoma.

TABLE 3.6

Differential diagnoses of acute angle closure

- All causes of an acute red eye
- Acute conjunctivitis
- Acute uveitis
- Neovascular glaucoma
- Foreign body

Primary congenital glaucoma is a rare condition. The diagnosis is critical, as treatment of the disease at an early stage gives a good prognosis and can prevent a lifetime of blindness. The diagnosis requires a high index of suspicion amongst those caring for pregnant women and newborn children.

Onset of congenital glaucoma is from birth to 2 years of age. However, many cases present at a later age with severe disease, particularly in developing countries.

The diagnosis requires a comprehensive eye examination, including measurement of IOP, examination of the optic disc and, if possible, examination of the angle of the eye, usually under sedation or anesthesia. Repeated examinations under anesthesia are the norm in the management of this disease.

Diagnostic signs. The optic disc and sclera are highly elastic in children. High IOP often causes rapid ocular enlargement and induces myopia. The size of the cornea is an important diagnostic sign. The corneal diameter should be 9–9.5 mm at birth, 9.5–10.5 mm at 6 months of age and 10.5–11.5 mm at 1 year. A measurement of 12 mm or more is considered abnormal. Stretching of the limbus produces tears in Descemet's membrane, called Haab's striae (Figure 3.29). The combination of a corneal diameter of 12 mm or more in the presence of Haab's striae is pathognomonic for congenital glaucoma.

IOP is lower in children than in adults but the IOP cut-off for adult glaucoma is usually applied.

Glaucomatous changes in the optic disc in children tend to manifest as a large CDR. Glaucoma should be suspected in an infant with a CDR greater than 0.3, particularly if the IOP is raised. An asymmetry

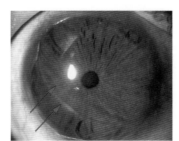

Figure 3.29 Haab's striae in congenital glaucoma (arrowed).

TABLE 3.7

Differential diagnoses of primary congenital glaucoma

- Megalo-cornea: an increased corneal diameter with no other signs of glaucoma
- Nasolachrymal duct obstruction: no signs of glaucoma
- Keratitis: a hazy cornea but without enlarged corneal diameters or raised intraocular pressure (IOP); other signs of inflammation may be present
- Metabolic storage disorders: hazy corneas with no other signs of glaucoma
- Intraocular tumor (e.g. retinoblastoma): raised IOP and hazy corneas

of CDR – especially in combination with an increased CDR or myopia in the eye with the raised IOP – is a strong indicator of congenital glaucoma.

Examination of the visual field is almost impossible in children under 5 years of age. Children find it difficult to perform conventional perimetry but do better on the frequency-doubling perimeter using its screening mode, which takes about a minute. Once they are old enough to cooperate, conventional automated perimetry can be performed.

Differential diagnoses of congenital glaucoma are listed in Table 3.7. Intraocular tumors can be diagnosed by the presence of new vessels on the iris; tumors should be evident on fundus examination or ultrasonography (if the media is hazy). A high index of suspicion is necessary.

Secondary glaucoma. The signs of glaucoma are the same in secondary glaucoma as in primary glaucoma. The diagnosis is made by finding a cause for the raised IOP or trabecular dysfunction on history taking or during the course of a comprehensive eye examination.

Common causes of secondary glaucoma include:

- pseudoexfoliation: pseudoexfoliative material obstructs the trabecular network and can be seen on the lens (see Figure 3.1, page 37)

- pigment dispersion: characterized by disruption of the iris pigment epithelium, deposition of pigment granules on the back of the cornea (Krukenberg's spindle), slit-like radial and mid-peripheral iris transillumination defects and dense pigmentation that obstructs the trabecular meshwork (Figure 3.30)
- trauma: blunt trauma can cause damage to the angle
- neovascularization of the iris caused by retinal ischemia in diabetes mellitus or central retinal vein occlusion (Figure 3.31)
- steroid use: usually topical steroids
- lens-induced glaucoma
- lenticular abnormalities, syndromes and tumors (in children).

Pseudoexfoliation is by far the most common cause of secondary glaucoma worldwide. However, as the signs of pseudoexfoliation can manifest after glaucoma diagnosis is made, epidemiological studies usually include pseudoexfoliation glaucoma in primary OAG.

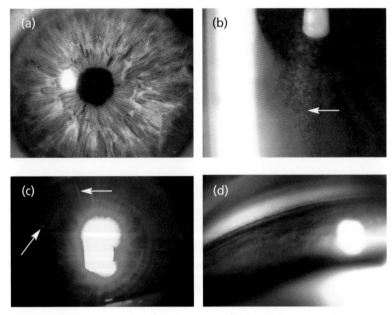

Figure 3.30 Pigment dispersion: (a) on the iris; (b) on the back of the cornea (Krukenberg's spindle); (c) mid-peripheral slit-like transillumination defects (arrowed spokes); (d) homogenous pigmentation of the trabecular meshwork.

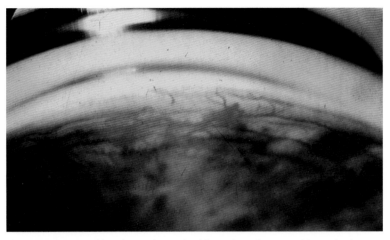

Figure 3.31 New blood vessels on the iris and angle caused by retinal ischemia.

Key points – diagnosis and clinical features

- Glaucoma is a common, potentially blinding disorder; diagnosis at an early stage, when intervention can alter the course of the disease and change the prognosis, is therefore preferable.
- Glaucoma can only be diagnosed after a comprehensive eye examination comprising measurement of intraocular pressure (IOP), gonioscopy and examination of the optic disc. This examination should be performed on all patients presenting to an ophthalmologist. If the optic disc is suspicious, visual field tests will confirm functional damage.
- No single glaucoma test (visual field or optic nerve imaging) should be interpreted in isolation. Structural and functional abnormalities should correlate. Where this is not the case, alternative tests should corroborate the initial finding.
- Primary open-angle glaucoma is a diagnosis of exclusion; the most common error is to mistake it for primary angle-closure glaucoma.
- Although a rare condition, primary congenital glaucoma must be detected and treated early to prevent a lifetime of blindness.

Managing a chronic disease such as glaucoma involves much more than prescribing medication or performing surgery. The goal of management of glaucoma is to improve health by:
- minimizing the impact (the burden of disease) on the patient
- reducing the risk factors for the development or progression of the glaucoma, in order to prevent visual impairment that would interfere with the patient's life
- minimizing the impact of treatment (side effects)
- encouraging adherence to therapy.

The state, rate of progression and risk factors for glaucoma must be re-evaluated regularly.

Minimizing the impact of glaucoma

The effects of early- and late-stage glaucoma are outlined in Table 4.1.

The early stages. Many people are more afraid of blindness than they are of cancer. Just being given a diagnosis of a potentially blinding disease can worsen health and create considerable anxiety and possibly depression.

Initial consultations. At the initial consultation the doctor must clearly explain the nature of glaucoma, the realistic prognosis and the rationale for the management plan. Empathy and reassurance can do much to allay fears and help a patient to take ownership of their disease and its management. Rarely can nothing positive be done or said during a medical consultation. Most patients do not recall much after being given bad news, so the initial conversation should be reinforced at subsequent visits until the doctor is certain the patient has an appropriate understanding of the condition.

It is not unusual for well-managed glaucoma to be stable over many years. It is just as important for the patient to know that their efforts with treatment are paying off with disease stability as it is for them to know if the disease has progressed.

TABLE 4.1

Effects of glaucoma

Early stages

- Anxiety about prognosis
- Increased awareness of physiological or minor pathological visual and ocular disturbances
- Reduction in contrast sensitivity

Later stages

- Injury through trauma brought about by scotomas
- Reduced reading ability
- Manifest reduction in the subjective visual field
- Reduction in standard (high-contrast) visual acuity
- Darkening of the subjective visual field
- Loss of visual fixation
- Loss of light perception

General problems at any stage

- Ocular pain or headaches from high intraocular pressure or the primary cause of secondary glaucoma
- Adverse reactions to glaucoma treatment

Explaining symptoms. Many systemic, visual and ocular disturbances that are usually ignored or disregarded can take on fearful new implications when someone has an eye disease such as glaucoma. Headache (especially retro-orbital), eye pain, epiphora (watery eyes), photopsias (flashes of light generated by retinal traction), shadows from vitreous floaters and presbyopia (reduced accommodation with increasing age) can all be misinterpreted as symptoms of glaucoma. The real causes of these symptoms and their significance need to be explained carefully.

Adapting to a reduction in contrast sensitivity. One of the visual changes in many eye diseases, including cataract and glaucoma, is a reduction in contrast sensitivity. This manifests in glaucoma as difficulty adapting to very bright or dark environments. Subjective glare disability in bright light and difficulty adjusting to dim light or dark conditions can have major effects on normal activities. Simple interventions such as correcting refractive errors with spectacles, the use of sunglasses and broad-brimmed hats, and installation of adequate home lighting can improve quality of life considerably.

Glaucoma and cataract become increasingly common with older age, thus it is not unusual for a patient to have both conditions in the same eye. The presence of glaucoma may increase the disability from cataract and reduce the maximum vision achievable from cataract removal. While decisions about cataract surgery in patients with glaucoma require good clinical judgment, the likely benefit of cataract surgery should not be dismissed just because glaucoma is also present.

The later stages. The visual fields of the two eyes overlap, and in the binocular visual field visual ability is determined by the vision in the better-seeing eye (see Chapter 2, page 27 and Figure 2.6). As scotomas enlarge and deepen, patients can experience difficulties seeing objects coming from the side, walking over uneven ground, and judging depth and distance. The results of glaucomatous visual field loss can include road traffic accidents, tripping over or bumping into objects, and falling up or down stairs. The injuries sustained (especially in an elderly person) can have a large impact.

Driving restrictions. Most driving licensing authorities require notification of the disease and impose restrictions relating to glaucoma and loss of peripheral vision. Many elderly people regard driving as an important connection to the wider community and are reluctant to do anything that might jeopardize the renewal of their driving license. Patients should be counseled about their obligations, and the danger of driving with visual field loss should be emphasized.

Improving the patient's immediate environment. Good lighting and contrast (particularly color contrast) can improve navigation around the home. Minimizing the difficulties posed by stairs, leveling uneven ground and installing hand rails can help reduce the risk of falls. Public authorities have an obligation to make public footpaths even and well lit.

Reading is highly valued by many people, and loss of reading ability is a source of fear for many patients with glaucoma. Reduced contrast sensitivity can be improved with even high-quality lighting. Mistracking from scotomas can be minimized by using a guide (such as a ruler) while reading.

The end stages of glaucoma are marked by loss of central visual acuity and fixation at light perception. Physical assistance becomes increasingly important in these stages. As with any disease of a special sense, maximizing the other senses can improve quality of life. It is particularly important to treat hearing and balance disorders in people with severe visual impairment.

Reducing risk factors

Reduction of intraocular pressure (IOP) has been proven to reduce the risk of both developing glaucoma and glaucoma progression, and it is the overwhelming focus of therapy.

Normal intraocular pressure. The IOP maintains the positions of the cornea, lens and retina within the eye. Normal values for IOP vary between populations but, usually, the mean IOP is 15–16 mmHg with a standard deviation (SD) of 2.5–3.0 mmHg. This means that the normal or 95% range (mean ± 2 SD) for IOP is 9–21 mmHg (in Korean and Japanese people, mean IOP is 14 mmHg with a SD of 2 mmHg). This does not mean that IOP below 21 mmHg cannot contribute to glaucoma; the risk of incident glaucoma and its progression increases continuously right through the IOP range. The precise pressure at which glaucoma will develop or progress depends on other factors, only some of which can be measured.

The aim of management is to prevent visual disability, not to stop the disease process or to lower IOP per se.

IOP is influenced by a number of factors (Table 4.2; Figure 4.1).

Controlling intraocular pressure. The ultimate aim when lowering IOP is to return it to the previous normal level or to the level of the contralateral normal eye – this is the pressure that the eye would have if glaucoma had not developed; however, often we do not know the normal eye pressure for that particular eye. For congenital glaucoma, the eye pressure may never have been normal. In these cases, we reduce

71

TABLE 4.2

Factors that influence intraocular pressure

Factor	Influence on intraocular pressure (IOP)	Impact
Posture*	IOP increases when supine	Large
Time of day*	IOP increases early morning	Large
Hydration	IOP increases when hydrated	Large
Central corneal thickness	IOP can be erroneously underestimated when the central corneal thickness is low	Variable
Blood pressure	IOP increases when systemic blood pressure is raised	Small

*See Figure 4.1.

the IOP by a percentage (e.g. 30–50%) or to a level referenced by the population IOP (e.g. 1–2 SD below the mean).

A single IOP reading may be misleading. Best practice in the clinical setting is to measure IOP at different times of day (if necessary, by scheduling patient visits at different times); any 'high' readings should be confirmed by repeat measurement.

Setting a target pressure. The Early Manifest Glaucoma Treatment (EMGT) study showed that a reduction in IOP of at least 25% reduced the proportion of participants whose glaucoma progressed over 5 years from 62% to 45%. In the Collaborative Initial Glaucoma Treatment Study (CIGTS), a 35% reduction of IOP by both medical and surgical treatment regimens decreased the proportion of participants in whom disease progressed to less than 15%.

Our current best guess for the IOP that will be commensurate with no subjective visual loss depends on the IOP sensitivity of the disease, the IOP tolerance of the optic nerve and life expectancy of the patient. A general rule for IOP targets based on the the average IOP of a normal person (the population mean pressure) is given in Table 4.3. We cannot know the IOP sensitivity of a patient's disease a priori, although glaucoma that occurs at higher IOPs tends to be more IOP sensitive. We can guess at the IOP tolerance of the optic nerve from the amount of

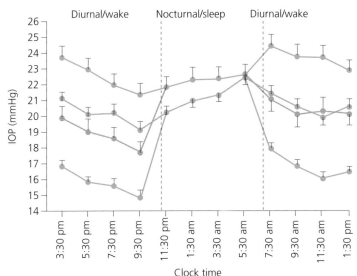

Figure 4.1 The effect of time and posture on intraocular pressure (IOP) in patients aged 40–78 years with newly diagnosed early glaucoma and age-matched controls with healthy eyes. In the same posture, IOP is usually highest in the early morning and lowest just before sleep. But IOP is always high supine compared with upright. This accentuates the difference between night and day IOPs. Reproduced with permission from Liu JH, Zhang X, Kripke DF, Weinreb RN. Twenty-four-hour intraocular pressure pattern associated with early glaucomatous changes. *Invest Ophthalmol Vis Sci* 2003;44:1586–90.

damage at diagnosis at the presenting IOP. Eyes with little damage despite long periods of high IOP tend to have a better prognosis for a given amount of IOP reduction.

While central vision is preserved, more advanced damage warrants more aggressive IOP lowering, partly because we assume a faster rate of progression and partly because further progression will have a greater impact on quality of life. Treatment guidelines suggest lowering IOP by:

- at least 20% in mild glaucoma (or 1 SD above the usual target)
- 30% in moderate glaucoma
- more than 40% in severe glaucoma (or 1 SD below the usual target).

TABLE 4.3

Target intraocular pressure for treatment on the basis of the pressure at which damage occurred

Pressure at which damage occurred	Target pressure
> 2 SD above population mean (i.e. > 21–22 mmHg)	Population mean (15–16 mmHg)
Up to 2 SD above population mean	1 SD below population mean (i.e. 12–13 mmHg).
At or below population mean	1–2 SD below population mean (i.e. 8–11 mmHg)

SD, standard deviation.

Lastly, the ability of glaucoma to destroy vision depends on life expectancy. Patients with long life expectancies usually warrant more aggressive treatment for a given disease state.

The target IOP is not always a fixed number, and regular monitoring is required to measure the rate of progression at target IOP (see Chapter 7).

It is not possible to medically lower IOP below the pressure in the episcleral veins. Doing so surgically risks the clinical syndrome of hypotony, which itself can cause substantial disability.

How to lower intraocular pressure

Intraocular pressure can be lowered by a variety of means, as detailed below. Medical treatments are discussed in more detail in Chapter 5, and laser and surgical treatments in Chapter 6.

Reverse any mechanism that will damage the trabecular meshwork.

- Prevent iridotrabecular contact in primary angle closure and angle-closure glaucoma by preventing pupil block (peripheral iridotomy) and moving the iris away from the trabecular meshwork (laser peripheral iridoplasty and lens extraction).
- Prevent secondary angle closure by treating the underlying cause (ischemic neovascularization, uveitis, aqueous misdirection, tumors).

Correct abnormal trabecular meshwork structure to improve function.

- Cut through trabecular tissue in congenital glaucoma (goniotomy, trabeculotomy).
- Break peripheral anterior synechiae in primary angle closure (goniosynechiolysis).

Improve aqueous outflow or reduce aqueous production.

- Increase uveoscleral outflow by application of topical prostaglandin analogs (PGAs: latanoprost, travoprost, bimatoprost, unoprostone). It should be noted that although the uveoscleral outflow pathway is not thought to have a major effect on IOP in normal eyes, enhancing uveoscleral outflow can dramatically reduce IOP in glaucoma.
- Improve trabecular outflow by argon or selective laser trabeculoplasty (ALT, SLT, respectively).
- Reduce aqueous production by application of topical β-blockers (timolol, levobunolol, carteolol, betaxolol).
- Reduce aqueous production, and possibly increase trabecular outflow, with α_2-agonist (brimonidine, apraclonidine).
- Reduce aqueous production with topical carbonic anhydrase inhibitors (dorzolamide, brinzolamide).

  Other treatments that have a role in improving trabecular outflow or reducing aqueous production but are used less often, mainly because of poor effect or adverse events, include:

- cholinergic agents (pilocarpine, carbachol) – increase trabecular outflow
- systemic or topical adrenergic agonists (dipivefrine, adrenaline/epinephrine) – reduce aqueous production
- systemic carbonic anhydrase inhibitors (acetazolamide, methazolamide, dichlorphenamide) – reduce aqueous production
- diode laser cyclophotocoagulation of the ciliary body – reduces aqueous production.

Bypass the trabecular meshwork by creating a fistula through the wall of the eye by trabeculectomy (including variants such as deep sclerectomy and other so-called 'non-penetrating' techniques) or implantation of drainage tubes. Antifibrosis agents often need to be used adjunctively to control postoperative closure of the fistula or its drainage into the venous/lymphatic system.

Minimizing adverse reactions

The best treatment is the least that achieves the most. For many people with open-angle glaucoma, a single drop of a PGA once a day may be all that is required. This class of drug usually has high efficacy and few side effects. Other people with glaucoma need multiple high-risk surgical procedures, which come with a large number of debilitating side effects and the IOP may remain higher than desired.

The key to judging the risk of adverse effects of treatments is to balance the likelihood of treatment success against the risk of adverse effects of the disease itself. For example, a patient who requires a simple eye drop regimen but receives high-risk surgery could suffer unnecessarily. Conversely, a patient who requires surgical treatment but receives only eye drops could become blind.

The benefit of a glaucoma treatment must also be balanced against the cost of the treatment, the costs of other treatments for glaucoma and other costs in the patient's life.

Managing conditions that may lead to glaucoma

Many people who have no evidence of glaucoma on examination nevertheless have one or more risk factors for the disease. Prophylactic intervention in these patients will depend on the estimated risk of glaucoma and subsequent visual disability.

Treatment decisions relating to conditions that almost always lead to glaucoma are easier. Examples include angle closure, angle neovascularization and extreme ocular hypertension (more than 5 standard deviations above the mean). Treatment decisions are more difficult where the risk is lower or unknown; for example, moderate ocular hypertension, narrow iridocorneal angles or patients with multiple systemic and ocular risk factors.

While each treatment decision needs to be made on an individual basis, patients in all risk categories need regular follow-up so that the presence or development of glaucoma can be determined. Monitoring is discussed in detail in Chapter 7.

Signs of glaucoma without collaborative/corroborative evidence

Sometimes a clear diagnosis of glaucoma cannot be made because of a lack of corroborative evidence. The appearance of the optic disc may suggest glaucomatous optic neuropathy, even though there is no evidence of progressive damage or impairment of visual function. Alternatively, a visual field defect may be present but with no ocular signs of glaucoma. Such glaucoma-like visual field defects have been reported in a variety of non-glaucomatous conditions, from myopia to other optic neuropathies such as anterior ischemic optic neuropathy.

Treatment decisions in these cases depend on the estimated risk of visual disability. Irrespective of intervention, regular follow-up is prudent unless the physician can be certain the findings are benign.

Control of intraocular pressure in the absence of glaucoma

The Ocular Hypertension Treatment Study examined the 5-year rate of glaucoma development in individuals with ocular hypertension with and without IOP-lowering treatment. The proportion of participants developing glaucomatous disc damage or field loss was approximately 4% in the treatment group vs 10% in the control group. Individual risk depended on age, IOP, central corneal thickness, and initial optic disc and visual field findings. However, in general, damage was rare and slow. Most recommendations now suggest not treating ocular hypertension unless risk is high.

Key points – principles of management

- The effects of a diagnosis of glaucoma vary over the different stages of the disease.
- The goal of management of glaucoma is to improve health by minimizing disability from disease and treatment.
- Estimates of rate of progression of visual field loss can be used to predict the progression of glaucoma.
- Rate of disease progression can usually be slowed by risk factor reduction – primarily the reduction of intraocular pressure.

Most patients with glaucoma are treated medically. Before embarking on any medical treatment, it is important to remember the key aims of preserving visual function and quality of life of the individual patient. Essentially, (functional) vision should outlast the patient. The aim is not to treat just intraocular pressure (IOP), the optic disc or visual field, but to treat the patient as a whole in order to provide maximum benefit with minimal side effects.

The target IOP can be defined as the highest IOP in a given eye at which no visually disabling nerve damage occurs; or, better still, the IOP at which health-related quality of life (with preserved vision and no side effects from treatment) is maximized. Keeping these concepts in mind will prevent over- or under-treatment. Further information on target IOP is given in Chapter 4 (pages 72–4 and Table 4.3).

Eye drop technique

The goal of medical treatment is to obtain 24-hour control of IOP with the minimum concentration and number of medications, as well as minimal local and systemic side effects. The correct instillation of eye drops should be demonstrated, and patients need to be encouraged to perform eyelid closure and punctal occlusion after instilling each medication (Figure 5.1).

Drug selection

Selection of the initial drug depends on the target IOP (see Chapter 4). Factors to keep in mind when prescribing a drug include:
- efficacy
- safety
- adherence to therapy
- persistence
- affordability.

Patient concordance and persistence with treatment are likely to be optimal when dosage is convenient, side effects are minimal and the

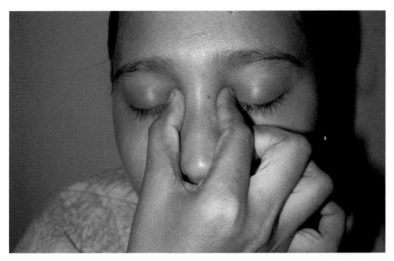

Figure 5.1 Eyelid closure and punctal occlusion following instillation of an eye drop.

drug is affordable. Introduction of fixed-combination treatments has helped to improve adherence and reduce costs.

Table 5.1 shows the available medications used to lower IOP in glaucoma with their mechanisms of action, time to peak effect and side effects.

Establishing efficacy. Once initiated, glaucoma therapy is usually life long, involves considerable expense and inconvenience, and has the potential for side effects. Accordingly, before initiating therapy, the physician must be sure of the diagnosis and reasonably sure that the medication will work. A unilateral drug trial will determine the efficacy of a single or combined therapy in one eye. The efficacy of the components of a fixed combination should be tested separately first, however.

Therapy is usually started in the eye with higher IOP and greater structural and functional damage. Fluctuation and peak IOPs are best assessed by 24-hour monitoring, but as this is impractical, 2- or 3-hourly measurements during the daytime can be made. If the drug achieves the target IOP, it is continued in that eye and treatment is started in the second eye.

TABLE 5.1

Drug treatments for glaucoma

Drug	Mechanism of action	Duration of action
Prostaglandin analogs • Latanoprost 0.005% • Bimatoprost 0.03% • Travoprost 0.004% • Unoprostone 0.15%	Increases uveoscleral outflow	24 hours
β-blockers • Timolol 0.25%, 0.5% • Levobunolol 0.25%, 0.5% • Betaxolol 0.25%, 0.5% • Carteolol 1%	Decreases aqueous production	12 hours
Carbonic anhydrase inhibitors (CAIs) *Systemic* Acetazolamide 250 mg *Topical* • Dorzolamide 2% • Brinzolamide 1%	Decreases aqueous production	6–8 hours

Systemic side effects	Local side effects	Peak effect and washout period

Skin rash
Skin pigmentation
Iris hyperchromia
	Reactivation of herpetic
	  keratitis
	Cystoid macular edema in
	  patients with a pseudophakic
	  or aphakic eye
		Peak effect:
		  6 weeks to
		  2 months
		Washout:
		  4–6 weeks

Bradycardia Hypotension Asthma Bronchospasm Dyspnea Impotence Insomnia Hypoglycemia	Allergic blepharoconjunctivitis Dry eye Corneal anesthesia	Both 4–6 weeks

Fatigue, malaise
Paresthesias of
  fingers and toes
Cramps
Diarrhea
Nephrolithiasis
  (calcium oxalate
  and calcium
  phosphate)
Renal failure
Acute leukopenia
Agranulocytosis
Aplastic anemia
Hemolytic anemia
Hypokalemia
Metabolic acidosis
Stevens–Johnson
  syndrome
Contraindicated
  in patients with
  'sulfa' allergy
	Conjunctival hyperemia
	Allergic reactions
	Blepharitis
	Burning/stinging sensation
	Irreversible corneal edema in
	  patients with compromised
	  endothelium (e.g. subclinical
	  Fuchs' dystrophy, post-surgical
	  changes)
		Peak effect:
		  72 hours
		Washout: 1 week

CONTINUED

TABLE 5.1 (CONTINUED)

Drug	Mechanism of action	Duration of action
Adrenergic agents α_2-adrenergic agonists: • Apraclonidine 0.5%, 1% • Brimonidine 0.2%, 0.15%	Decreases aqueous production, partially increases uveoscleral outflow	8 hours
Other (less used) adrenergic agonists: *Systemic* • Adrenaline (epinephrine) • Dipivefrine *Topical* • Epinephrine borate 0.5%, 1% • Dipivefrine 0.1%	Decreases aqueous production and increases outflow facility	8 hours
Cholinergics (miotics) • Pilocarpine 1%, 2%, 4%	Increases trabecular outflow by constricting longitudinal ciliary body muscle and opening trabecular meshwork	6–8 hours

Systemic side effects	Local side effects	Peak effect and washout period
Drowsiness Headache Dry mouth Marked fatigue Crosses blood–brain barrier **Absolutely contraindicated in patients taking monoamine oxidase inhibitor**	Allergic conjunctivitis	Peak effect: 2 weeks (stabilizes at 6 weeks) Washout: 4–6 weeks
Headache Nervousness Tachycardia Arrhythmia Hypertension Dry mouth Drowsiness	Mydriasis Lid retraction Adrenochrome deposits Allergic follicular conjunctivitis Cystoid macular edema in aphakia	Peak effect: 2 weeks (stabilizes at 6 weeks) Washout: 1 week
Increased sweating Salivation Bradycardia Tachycardia	Miosis Accommodative spasm Iris cysts Anterior subcapsular lens opacity Lacrimation	Peak effect: within 3 hours Washout: 1 week

CONTINUED

TABLE 5.1 (CONTINUED)

Drug	Mechanism of action	Duration of action
Hyperosmotic agents Mannitol Oral glycerol	Increases osmolality of blood, thus drawing aqueous from vitreous	8 hours

Adapted from Parikh RS, Parikh SR, Navin S et al. Practical approach to medical management of glaucoma. *Indian J Ophthalmol* 2008;56:223–30.

If the drug fails to reduce IOP by at least 15% from baseline, or produces intolerable side effects, it is not prescribed, and a unilateral drug trial should be started with a second drug option. If the first drug does reduce IOP by more than 15% from baseline but not to the target IOP level, the trial has nevertheless established that the medication works. Either a second medication can be added, or treatment can be switched to a new medication. Usually the tested drug is kept as a reserve medicine to be used in combination if other options do not provide adequate control of IOP. A management algorithm for glaucoma, adapted from guidelines issued by the South & East Asia Glaucoma Interest Group (SEAGIG) and the National Institute for Health and Clinical Excellence (NICE, UK) is shown in Figure 5.2.

Systemic side effects	Local side effects	Peak effect and washout period
Nausea and vomiting		Mannitol: peak effect: within 1 hour
Circulatory overload – congestive heart failure, pulmonary edema, hyponatremia, dehydration		
Cerebrospinal fluid acidosis in patients with poor renal function		
Caution required in patients with cardiac, renal or hepatic disease		
Oral glycerol contraindicated in patients with diabetes		

Disadvantages of unilateral drug trials. Although nothing acute or significantly detrimental is likely to happen during the time it takes to perform a unilateral trial, many patients (and doctors) are uncomfortable with treating only one eye, particularly if the baseline IOP is high. The duration of the trial depends on the drug: sometimes a trial lasts only a few hours (cholinergics) or days (alpha agonists) but usually about a month to 6 weeks (β-blockers and prostaglandin analogs [PGAs]). If the glaucoma is advanced and the IOP is very high, an alternative is to perform a reverse therapeutic trial. In this scenario, both eyes are treated and more than one medication may be initiated; when the target IOP is reached, the medications are reduced one by one (in one eye) until the optimal treatment is found, i.e. the minimum drug

85

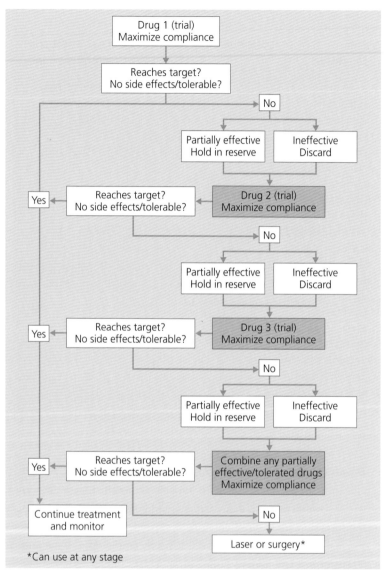

Figure 5.2 Management algorithm (see text for details) adapted from national guidelines: NICE Clinical Guideline 85. *Management of chronic open angle glaucoma and ocular hypertension.* London: National Collaborating Centre for Acute Care, 2009. www.nice.org.uk/nicemedia/pdf/CG85FullGuideline.pdf SEAGIG Asia Pacific Glaucoma Guidelines. Sydney: South East Asia Glaucoma Interest Group, 2003–4. www.seagig.org/toc/APGGuidelinesNMview.pdf

combination that maintains target IOP. As the peak effect and washout period of systemic acetazolamide are minimal, we prefer to use this drug when the situation demands reduction of IOP in the contralateral eye while we are waiting to assess the effects of the unilateral trial. Discontinuing systemic acetazolamide 72 hours before the next follow-up allows the effect of the eye drop to be assessed in one eye without too much risk to the other eye.

If the patient is unable to return within 4–6 weeks to assess the results of the unilateral trial, treatment in both eyes should be started and a reverse trial performed.

First-line treatment. The drug class with the greatest efficacy to side effect ratio is the PGAs. PGAs that can be administered as a once-daily dose such as latanoprost 0.005%, bimatoprost 0.03% or travoprost 0.004% are preferred. Some patients may not respond to one particular PGA but may respond to another. Therefore, if a PGA does not work it is worthwhile trying another.

Before the advent of PGAs, topical β-blockers were the most widely prescribed treatment class. Compared with PGAs, topical β-blockers are less effective and carry risks of serious systemic side effects. β-blockers are now the principal second-line agents, either as monotherapy or in fixed or unfixed combinations. Many PGAs are still under patent and command a large price premium. In price-sensitive markets, β-blockers are still prescribed as first-line treatment, but this is likely to change as PGAs lose patent rights.

Systemic β-blockers can achieve 80% of the effect of topical eye drops on IOP. If the patient is already taking systemic β-blockers for hypertension, topical β-blockers are unlikely to reduce IOP significantly and may not be appropriate as first-line treatment in these patients. Elderly patients with even mild chronic obstructive pulmonary disease (COPD) can have serious exacerbations on β-blockers. They would do better with an α-agonist such as brimonidine P 0.15% or a topical carbonic anhydrase inhibitor (CAI) rather than timolol.

If IOP reduction of 30% or more is required, a PGA can be combined with a β-blocker, α_2-adrenergic agent or CAI. If the PGA does not achieve the target IOP, or there is a cost issue, a combination of a β-blocker with an α_2-adrenergic agent such as brimonidine P 0.15% or a topical CAI may suffice. Drug combinations have made life easier, but each component must first be shown to be effective individually.

Generally, the IOP cannot be lowered below the episcleral venous pressure. Once the IOP is lowered by the first medication, the amount it can be further lowered (to the episcleral pressure) is less for the second medication. Accordingly, the second medication will seem to perform worse than if it were the first drug used.

Maximum tolerated medical therapy

If the target IOP is not reached with the first drug, further drugs may be added or substituted depending on the target IOP required. There is no consensus on how many drugs can be used. Maximal tolerated medical therapy can be defined as the minimum number and concentration of tolerable drugs (within the combination of different classes of medications) that provides maximum lowering of IOP. Medical treatment should be tailored to the individual patient.

Fixed-combination drops can improve adherence and decrease costs. The effectiveness of the individual components of the fixed dose should have been demonstrated previously in separate unilateral trials. Fixed-dose combinations include:

- a PGA and a β-blocker (bimatoprost and timolol, latanoprost and timolol, travoprost and timolol)
- an α_2-agonist and a β-blocker (brimonidine and timolol)
- a CAI and a β-blocker (brinzolamide and timolol, dorzolamide and timolol)
- a cholinergic and a β-blocker (pilocarpine and timolol).

Patients find some formulations more comfortable than others; if this causes problems with adherence then a change of brand may be considered. If glaucoma continues to progress despite maximum medical therapy, non-medical therapies should be considered (see Chapter 6).

Side effects and contraindications

Table 5.1 shows the reported side effects of the common anti-glaucoma drugs. Table 5.2 lists the major contraindications that affect glaucoma management.

TABLE 5.2

Drug contraindications that affect glaucoma management

- Topical β-blockers are contraindicated in patients with bronchial asthma, congestive heart failure or heart block.
- Topical β-blockers may mask symptoms of hypoglycemia in patients with brittle diabetes and may aggravate myasthenia gravis.
- Patients taking systemic β-blockers may derive only minimal additional benefit from topical β-blockers.
- α-adrenergic agents such as brimonidine are contraindicated in patients taking monoamine oxidase inhibitors.
- A history of sulfonamide allergy can contraindicate the use of oral acetazolamide.
- A history of herpetic disease or uveitis may contraindicate the use of topical prostaglandin analogs.
- A history of corneal endothelial disease may contraindicate the use of topical carbonic anhydrase inhibitors.

β-blockers should be avoided in patients with asthma or heart block. Many older patients can develop bronchospasm and may feel much better once a β-blocker is stopped.

PGAs should be used cautiously in patients with a history of inflammatory glaucoma, herpetic keratitis or cystoid macular edema with a compromised posterior capsule. Before initiating therapy, patients should be made aware of the side effects of PGAs, which include elongation and hyperpigmentation of lashes and iris hyperchromia, particularly if the therapy is to be used in just one eye.

Topical CAIs should be used cautiously in patients with poor corneal endothelial status, as these agents can worsen corneal edema. α_2-Agonists can cross the blood–brain barrier and are absolutely contraindicated in infants and in patients who are taking monoamine oxidase inhibitors. α_2-Agonists also cause drowsiness, which can have a major effect on the patient's quality of life. This side effect can be decreased by using punctal occlusion and eyelid closure. Oral CAIs should not be used for a long duration without the consent of the patient's physician.

Medical management of special glaucoma subtypes

Primary angle-closure glaucoma. First-line management for primary angle closure and primary angle-closure glaucoma is laser iridotomy. In general, primary angle-closure glaucoma requires closer monitoring than primary open-angle glaucoma. After iridotomy has achieved an angle open to at least 180 degrees, medical management should be the same as for primary open-angle glaucoma. If the angle does not open, other angle-opening measures should be considered such as laser iridoplasty or lens extraction and goniosynechialysis.

The effect of PGAs is inversely proportional to the degree of the closed angle, and is minimal in a totally closed angle.

If a patient is taking pilocarpine, a PGA may not have as much of an effect on IOP, and other medications should be considered.

Primary congenital glaucoma requires surgical management; medical management can be used to stabilize IOP before surgery and as adjunctive treatment following surgery. Medical management has a larger role to play in secondary congenital glaucomas.

There is no widespread experience with the use of common anti-glaucoma medications in children, and all drugs must be used with care. No glaucoma medicines are specifically approved for use in children. It is best to use the lowest concentration of medication available, for example 0.25% timolol rather than 0.5%. α-Agonists such as brimonidine, which can cross the blood–brain barrier and can cause apnea, are contraindicated in children under 2 years of age. Children must be monitored for side effects such as somnolence. Punctal occlusion must be used, and the parents/carers warned about potential side effects.

Key points – medical treatment

- The goal of treatment is preservation of the patient's vision. This means treating the patient as a whole, not just the intraocular pressure (IOP), optic disc or visual field.
- Estimate the target IOP range.
- Choose the drug most likely to control the IOP with minimal effect on quality of life.
- Establish that the drug is working, preferably in a unilateral trial.
- Do not use an ineffective drug; substitute rather than add medications.
- Fixed-dose combinations can improve adherence and decrease costs, but they must be considered in terms of their individual components.
- If required, obtain a diurnal curve of IOP.
- Monitor the patient's IOP, iridocorneal angle, optic disc and visual field on a regular basis.

Laser trabeculoplasty

Laser trabeculoplasty (LTP) involves the application of laser energy to the trabecular meshwork. When successful, it enhances the aqueous outflow and lowers intraocular pressure (IOP); it is particularly effective when used as initial treatment. The mechanism is likely to be a combination of mechanical and biological effects of the laser on the trabecular meshwork. LTP is usually performed in patients with ocular hypertension or open-angle glaucoma. Its effect may be pronounced in pseudoexfoliation or pigment dispersion syndromes. LTP can also be used as an adjunct to medical management of the patient with open angles, is a quick outpatient procedure and is less invasive than incisional surgery.

LTP seems to have a greater IOP-lowering effect in patients with more pigmented trabecular meshworks (e.g. pseudoexfoliation). Such patients (and those with raised IOP, and open angles after cataract removal) are at high risk for functional damage and are therefore probably good candidates for primary LTP. LTP is generally not used in angle-closure, juvenile or congenital glaucoma.

In a compliant patient, LTP is best regarded as equivalent to topical medications. The amount of IOP lowering can vary from dramatic to inconsequential. The best indication is the effect in the contralateral eye. The duration of effect of LTP also varies widely. In general, successful LTP lasts for 2–5 years. After application of topical anesthesia to the conjunctiva, laser treatment is delivered through a slit lamp using a gonioscope-type contact lens. Two types of laser are used for LTP.

Argon laser trabeculoplasty (ALT), which has been in use for some 30 years, creates a small coagulative pit in the trabecular meshwork. Side effects include transiently raised IOP and inflammation, which are treated prophylactically. ALT is associated with efficacy similar to that achieved with timolol, but effects decrease with time. The procedure can be repeated if required, although re-treatments increase the risk of raised IOP and the need for emergency surgery.

Selective laser trabeculoplasty (SLT) is a newer procedure, similar to ALT and delivered in a similar fashion, using a Q-switched neodynium:yttrium-aluminum-garnet (Nd:YAG) laser. It applies about 100-fold less energy than the argon laser, and as a consequence local side effect rates are fewer. It also does not cause coagulative necrosis to the trabecular meshwork. Results with SLT appear to be similar to those with ALT, but the advantage of SLT is its repeatability.

Laser cycloablation
The aim of this treatment is to reduce aqueous production by applying laser to the ciliary tissue that produces it. It is usually used as a supplemental treatment to drainage surgery (see below) or in eyes with advanced secondary glaucoma.

Laser peripheral iridotomy
Laser peripheral iridotomy (LPI) uses laser energy to make a small hole in the iris (usually under the upper lid where it will cause no visual disturbance). It is most often performed to relieve pupil block in primary angle closure, where aqueous pressure in the posterior chamber of the eye pushes the iris forward, obstructing the trabecular meshwork.

Laser peripheral iridoplasty
In iridoplasty, laser spots are applied circumferentially to the far peripheral iris to cause contraction and thinning. This can be beneficial in both acute and chronic forms of primary angle closure.

Surgery
Surgery is usually considered if glaucoma continues to progress despite maximum medical therapy. Indications for surgery as a primary intervention include:
- socioeconomic factors
- younger age with potentially longer duration of disease
- disease status in both eyes
- presence of visually disabling cataract
- general health of the patient.

93

It may not be appropriate to operate on an 85-year-old person with advanced glaucoma in one eye and very early glaucoma in another eye, or a 45-year-old person with terminal malignancy. The decision must be tailored to the individual patient. Intervention is undertaken only after a detailed discussion of risks, benefits and patient preferences.

There are three types of surgery performed in glaucoma.

- Surgery to lower IOP by draining aqueous out of the eye, which can be used for any subtype of glaucoma.
- Surgery to lower IOP by cutting into the iridocorneal angle. This can be very successful but only in congenital glaucoma.
- Surgery to open the iridocorneal angle to allow better access of the aqueous to the trabecular meshwork. This is performed in primary angle-closure glaucoma as well as primary angle closure.

Drainage surgery. There are two main forms of drainage surgery: trabeculectomy and tube surgery.

Trabeculectomy creates a guarded fistula through the superior corneo-limbus under a scleral flap. In the early postoperative period, the tension on the flap from sutures controls the aqueous outflow and therefore IOP. After surgery, fibroblasts from Tenon's capsule (an immune-reactive tissue layer that lies between the sclera and conjunctiva) proliferate and migrate towards the scleral flap, trying to seal the flap shut with collagenous scar tissue. When trabeculectomy is successful, the scar tissue prevents excessive drainage in steady state or from trauma, and protects the overlying conjunctiva from hydrostatic pressure. It does not close the scleral flap or reduce the hydraulic conductivity of the surrounding tissues. Steady state IOP depends on aqueous production, the area of sub-Tenon's drainage (known as the bleb) and the rate of outflow from the bleb onto the extraocular veins and lymphatics. Excessive scarring is the main cause of failure of trabeculectomy. Antifibrotic agents including mitomycin-C and 5-fluorouracil are frequently applied to the Tenon's capsule during surgery to reduce the activity of Tenon's fibroblasts. The effects from these agents can last many years. Non-penetrating surgery is a variant of trabeculectomy that differs in some technical aspects.

Tube surgery has the same intent as trabeculectomy, but is executed by placing a silicone tube in the anterior chamber (or sometimes through the pars plana into the vitreous cavity) to drain aqueous to a plate placed under the posterior Tenon's capsule between the extraocular muscles. The posterior Tenon's capsule is much thicker, so a large plate (172–450 mm^2) is required to prevent scarring down of the bleb. While there is less ability to control IOP postoperatively with tube surgery, the posterior placement of the plate and the scar-resistant tube make it a more robust surgical solution when risk of trabeculectomy failure or complication is high.

IOP-lowering angle surgery. Abnormal iridocorneal angle anatomy in congenital glaucoma led surgeons to believe that raised IOP was caused by a membrane covering the trabecular meshwork. Goniotomy and trabeculotomy can be performed to cut through the trabecular meshwork from the inside and outside of the eye, respectively. While the pathological features of iridocorneal angle maldevelopment in congenital glaucoma are far more complicated than first thought, this surgery can safely and effectively lower IOP for many decades. In some cases, a trabeculotomy and trabeculectomy can be performed in one operation. Unfortunately, goniotomy and trabeculotomy do not work in adult glaucoma.

Angle-opening surgery. Although cataract extraction with intraocular lens implantation has separate visual indications, it can dramatically deepen the anterior chamber and open the iridocorneal angle. This is because an artificial intraocular lens is less than 1 mm thick compared with a crystalline lens, which is 3.5–5.5 mm thick in older people.

Goniosynechialysis surgery opens the iridocorneal angle by physically breaking peripheral anterior synechiae (PAS). It requires a direct view of the angle structures through a surgical gonioprism. It can also be performed without direct view by injecting hyper-dense viscoelastic substances into the angle to push back the iris, but this procedure is not as well controlled.

For appositional angle closure caused by the pressure of aqueous, LPI is the usual treatment of choice. However, the procedure can also be performed as a surgical iridectomy.

Key points – laser and surgical treatment

- There are two types of laser trabeculoplasty: argon laser trabeculoplasty (ALT) and selective laser trabeculopasty (SLT). Results are similar with both types but SLT can be repeated if necessary.
- Laser peripheral iridotomy uses laser energy to make a small hole in the iris, usually to relieve pupil block in primary angle closure.
- Surgery should be considered if glaucoma continues to progress despite maximum medical therapy.
- Drainage surgery can be used for any type of glaucoma; trabeculectomy or tube surgery is performed to lower the intraocular pressure (IOP) by draining aqueous out of the eye.
- IOP-lowering angle surgery is a successful technique for congenital glaucoma.
- Angle-opening surgery, which allows better access of the aqueous to the trabecular meshwork, can be performed in patients with primary angle-closure glaucoma and primary angle closure.

The key to prevention of blindness from this chronic and slowly progressive disease is careful monitoring for progression. Such monitoring is performed by repeating the comprehensive eye examination (or some key parts of it as indicated) (see Chapter 3, page 35), as well as appropriate investigations, at regular intervals.

In this context, it is important to reiterate the goals of glaucoma management: to preserve vision and prevent loss of quality of life from the disease. The main principle of management is not to treat findings such as raised intraocular pressure (IOP), optic disc changes, signs of damage on imaging, or even visual field changes, in isolation. Information obtained from the history, examination and investigations should be used to treat any clear, present or future threat to this objective.

A real problem with the management of glaucoma is the long duration of the disease and the relatively slow rate of progression. It can be difficult to conceptualize the change in signs over many years, and impossible to remember the appearance of the optic disc from one year to the next. Accurate recording of structure, function and risk factors is therefore essential, as these recordings give an overview of the progress of the condition since diagnosis. It is vital to use this information in conjunction with the risk factor status to project potential future progress against life expectancy.

Even if treated, glaucoma will progress in many patients if they are followed up for long enough. Thus, the most important question to ask is not whether the glaucoma is progressing, but how quickly it is progressing (the rate of progression).

Rates of progression

We now know that in some patients glaucoma will progress slowly – perhaps only two or three times the normal aging rate – and often there will not be any significant risk of the condition becoming disabling during their lifetime. On the other hand, in a significant minority –

perhaps 15–20% – the condition will progress at 20–30 times the normal aging rate; in these cases, progression is so rapid the patient is at significant risk of becoming disabled in as little as 5–10 years. When IOPs are very high, bilateral blindness can occur within a couple of years. Thus, a patient whose condition is progressing rapidly must be managed differently from one whose condition is stable or progressing slowly. It is therefore important to establish the rate of progression soon after initial diagnosis, and to determine whether this is likely to put visual function at risk during that patient's expected lifetime. While there are no firm rules, it is clear that those with rapidly progressing disease who are in danger of reaching disability within, for instance, 7 years must be identified in a fraction of that time (e.g. in 2 or maybe 3 years at most), so that the downwards course can be arrested in a timely way.

Frequency of follow-up

Follow-up should be scheduled at regular intervals, the frequency of which depends on several factors. When change is suspected, more examinations are performed over a shorter period of time. In early stable disease, tests should be performed every 6–12 months, whereas every 2–4 months is more appropriate for unstable or more severe disease. If the clinical status changes, interim visits will be required until stability is achieved again.

The factors that determine the frequency of visits include:
- state (severity) of glaucoma
- rate of progression
- risk factors for accelerated progression, including higher IOP, optic disc hemorrhage and pseudoexfoliation syndrome
- initiation or change of treatment
- age
- general health status.

State of disease

Functional defects. Glaucoma state is probably best assessed by measuring the impact of binocular visual loss on functional abilities. We are unable to do this accurately or reliably, so at present the severity of disease is judged primarily by functional changes (field defects) on automated perimetry. Early defects generally require less frequent follow-up than moderate or advanced defects (Figure 7.1).

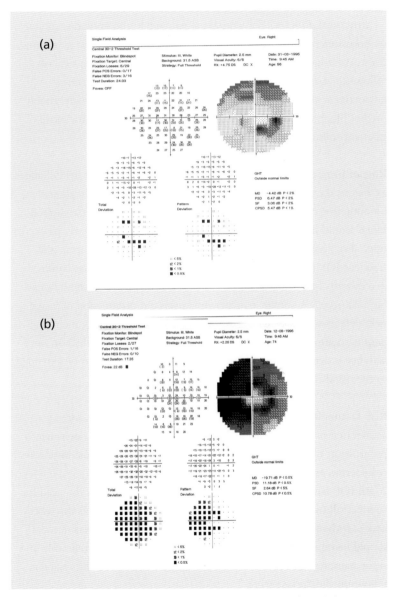

Figure 7.1 Automated perimetry printout of: (a) an early field defect; (b) an advanced field defect.

A defect that is close to, or involves, the fixation point (as in Figure 7.1b) requires close and frequent monitoring. Binocular field loss is more important than uniocular loss.

Structural damage. Glaucomatous damage in the optic disc alone, without functional defects in the visual field (pre-perimetric glaucoma), does not ordinarily necessitate the same frequency (or intensity) of follow-up as functional defects. Exceptions include optic disc hemorrhage and defects of the nerve fiber layer (NFL), which reliably predict functional deficits and therefore indicate the need for more frequent follow-up.

Rate of progression is determined by optic disc and visual field changes, as well as the level of IOP. A 60-year-old patient with early glaucoma, no optic disc changes, stable visual fields and IOP within the desired range would be followed up on a routine 6-monthly or yearly basis. An optic disc hemorrhage would trigger a visual field examination and frequent IOP measurements. Follow-up would be scheduled within 2–3 months but would return to a routine schedule once stability had been achieved. A similar patient with suspected progression of visual field defects would be called in for repeat visual field assessment and another comprehensive eye examination within 2–3 months but, once stability is demonstrated, the interval between visits would be extended to the usual routine schedule.

Risk factors for progression. Patients showing risk factors for accelerated progression need closer observation, either to determine if progression rate is changing or to change therapy. The most important risk factors are a rising IOP or an optic disc hemorrhage.

An IOP within the target range for the patient indicates the need for routine follow-up, but this also depends on other factors, as discussed above. If the IOP is higher than the stated target range, measurement should be repeated and confirmed at the same visit (and preferably at a subsequent follow-up). If changes are made to the treatment regimen, follow-up should be earlier.

An optic disc hemorrhage is a sign of nerve stress and is often

followed by worsening disc damage and/or visual field loss. It is the primary reason for examining the disc at every visit. Its appearance should initiate a re-evaluation of a patient's management plan.

Initiation or change of treatment should result in more frequent follow-up. For example, if a new drug is added for one eye, the effect can usually be estimated at a 2-week follow-up and determined fully after 4–6 weeks before reverting to the routine schedule of assessment.

Age. All things being equal, glaucoma is likely to have a greater impact on quality of life in a young patient than in someone older. A younger patient with an early visual field defect should be monitored and treated more aggressively than an older patient with a more limited life span. However, it should be noted that older age is itself a risk factor for more rapid progression.

General health and life expectancy have a substantial effect on the degree to which the patient is monitored and treated; this applies to any slowly progressive condition, not just glaucoma. A healthy 60-year-old person with early stable disease would be seen every 6–12 months. An 80-year-old person with advanced unstable glaucoma and a comorbid terminal illness would be monitored at the same intervals, not more intensively. Interventions for a progressive chronic disease like glaucoma are clearly more appropriate in someone with a long life expectancy who will ultimately be affected functionally by the disease. By contrast, judgment has to be made as to whether a person who is terminally ill, for example, or whose general health is not good should go through unnecessary surgery and the risks of complication, when he or she may not be functionally affected by the disease during his or her anticipated lifetime.

Estimating life expectancy. It is important to be able to estimate the life expectancy of a patient. Many ophthalmologists are (quite naturally) uncomfortable with integrating this element into their decision-making process and consider it impossible to assess the life expectancy of individual patients (although this is clearly not the case, as the life insurance industry accurately undertakes such assessments by taking into account factors such as smoking, alcohol consumption, general health and likely hereditary factors). As an extreme example, who is likely to live longer (and therefore need more careful follow-up and more aggressive treatment): a 75-year-old chronic smoker who has already had two heart attacks and whose parents died at 70 years of age, or a 75-year-old non-smoker in good general health whose parents lived beyond 85 years of age? Given the same stage of the disease, the latter patient would be monitored more frequently and is likely to merit more aggressive treatment.

Follow-up examinations

It is best to perform a comprehensive eye examination and investigations at each routine follow-up visit. When extra visits are required, the examination can be individualized and some specific steps may be omitted. As already discussed, progression is diagnosed by a combination of history, examination and investigations. A single finding or the results of an isolated investigation are not reliable.

Slit-lamp examination should be performed at every visit, to check for signs of inflammation, pseudoexfoliation, pigment dispersion etc. In patients with diabetes or retinal disease, the undilated pupillary margin should be examined for neovascularization.

Intraocular pressure should be measured at each visit. If progression is suspected on the basis of optic disc or visual field changes, or the effect of a new medication is being assessed, multiple IOP readings may be required. Such measurements are made either on the same day or at different times of the day at different visits (see page 40).

If the disease is progressing as expected according to the optic disc and visual field parameters, a 24-hour profile of the patient's IOP (usually obtained at 3-hourly intervals) may be required.

Gonioscopy should ideally be performed on a yearly basis. A previously documented open angle is not immune to angle closure as a result of pupillary block or lens-induced changes. Gonioscopy should be undertaken earlier if:

- the IOP increases and/or if progression (disc or field) is suspected
- other pathology (causing neovascularization) is suspected
- usual indications for such assessment exist (e.g. trauma to the eye).

In the course of pigment dispersion, pseudoexfoliative or uveitic glaucoma, the appearance of the trabecular meshwork can provide important information.

Gonioscopy is mandatory after any intervention to alter angle configuration (laser iridotomy or iridoplasty). Pilocarpine drops, which are used as an adjunct to such procedures, constrict the pupil and can artifactually open the angle. By relaxing the zonules and moving the lens forward, they can also close the angle. The effect of intervention should therefore be assessed after the effect of the eye drops has worn off (usually 48 hours).

Stereoscopic optic disc examination (preferably after dilatation of the pupil) should be performed at all regular visits. The optic disc should be specifically examined for a disc hemorrhage at every visit. Stereoscopic optic disc photographs with a 30-degree field of view should be obtained at a frequency that allows disc changes to be detected in a timely manner. A dilated examination of the fundus is also required to exclude retinal pathology as a cause of progressive visual field defects.

Documentation of disc appearance. Stereophotography of the optic disc is the gold standard to detect progression of optic disc changes. The most recent stereophotographs should be compared with those obtained at baseline and follow-up visits (Figure 7.2). A less accurate method is to note changes in diagrams and/or clinical descriptions.

Signs of structural progression. Recognizing change is useful for diagnosis as well as for the detection of progression. Identification of any of the signs described as diagnostic of the disease (see Chapter 3) indicates progression. Such signs include progressive loss of the neuroretinal rim, increased cup-to-disc ratio (a surrogate measure of rim loss, better measured as a rim-to-disc ratio), new rim notch or acquired pit.

Unlike a congenital pit, an acquired pit is caused by the disease and develops during its course. Changes in the positions of blood vessels are an important clue to underlying rim loss and can be detected early by

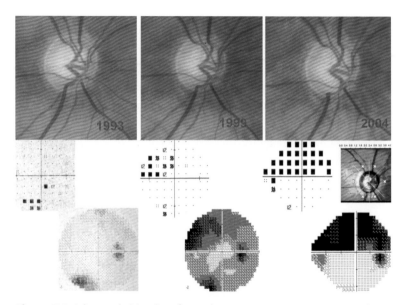

Figure 7.2 Advanced vision loss from glaucoma over an 11-year period. Vision was normal in 1993 but in a typical pattern of damage, the inferior rim of the optic nerve head is lost first. By 1999, the inferior neural rim has lost half its tissue and the overlying blood vessels have dropped down to the new rim edge. A dense scotoma is seen in the corresponding upper nasal visual field, although the most central part of the vision is still normal. By 2004, almost all the inferior rim has been lost. The change in vessel position is very obvious and the patient is now blind in the entire upper part of the visual field including fixation.

comparison of serial photographs. Disc hemorrhage and increasing parapapillary atrophy are also important signs (Figure 7.3).

The photographs should also be examined for loss of the bright–dark–bright striations of the NFL (see Figure 3.22, page 54) or the presence of a new wedge defect (see Figure 3.23, page 54), as well as for worsening of any such existing defects.

Imaging techniques. Although clinical examinations of the optic disc, drawings and clinical notes are useful to document disease state, they are of limited use for detecting the progression of disease. Even

gold-standard assessment by serial stereophotography is limited by

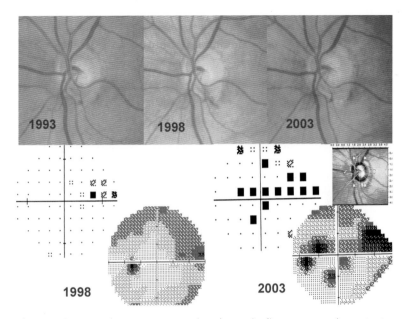

Figure 7.3 Hemorrhages on or crossing the optic disc are a very important prognostic sign of glaucoma progression. In 1993, the otherwise normal optic nerve has a residuum of an optic disc hemorrhage at the superior temporal disc margin. In 1998, another hemorrhage is visible, this time inferotemporally, although vision loss is minimal. By 2003, a deep notch has formed in the inferior neural rim with corresponding vision loss across the visual field just above the midline. A more subtle loss of the superior neural rim has caused a smaller area of inferior vision loss, but its location at fixation is a serious threat to vision.

differences in quality, magnification, focus and color, together with the subjectivity arising from the inherent skill of the physician. Modern imaging techniques attempt to address these limitations and have a major role in the detection of early disease progression. In the early stages of glaucoma, progression is usually best determined by techniques that examine structure.

The Heidelberg retinal tomogram (HRT) is a confocal scanning laser ophthalmoscope that generates a series of cross-sectional measurements of reflectivity through the semi-transparent neuroretinal tissues of the optic disc. These measurements allow the position of the surface of the NFL as it runs into the optic disc to be estimated. HRT has the longest track record in this area, with several programs that assess serial measurements for a decrease in surface height, indicating progression (Figure 7.4). Graphical trend analysis depicts normalized

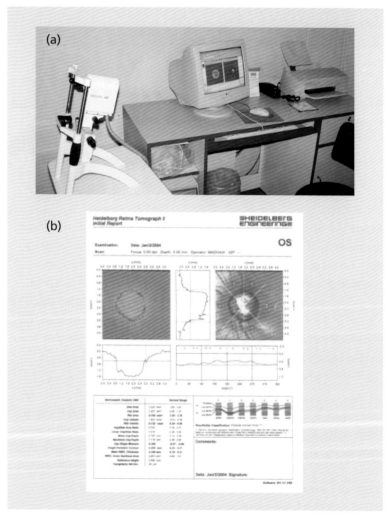

Figure 7.4 (a) The Heidelberg retinal tomography machine and (b) its usual printout in a patient with glaucoma. Glaucoma is indicated by the red crosses and exclamation mark (yellow) on the printout, as well as by the bar diagram.

changes of parameters reported by the HRT from baseline. A
downward trend in three consecutive examinations suggests change
(Figure 7.5a). Topographic change analysis compares the topography
in discrete areas of successive images, called superpixels. Change
probability maps show areas of statistically significant change over
three consecutive examinations. Areas of progression are shown in red,
while those that have improved are shown in green (Figure 7.5b). This
program eliminates operator-dependent marking of the optic disc
margin. Recent developments allow probability analysis for the depth
and size of change to be made. According to Professor Balawantry

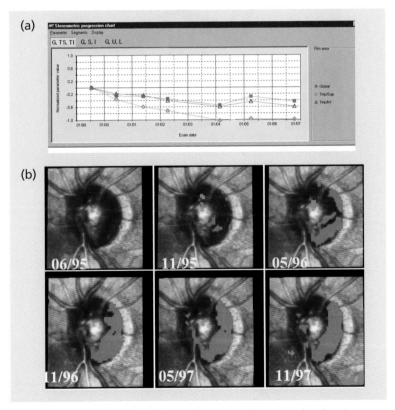

Figure 7.5 (a) Trend analysis by Heidelberg retinal tomography, showing a
downward trend that indicates worsening of disease status. (b) Topographic
change analysis; the increase in the area colored red indicates a loss of tissue.
Reproduced courtesy of Professor Balwantray Chauhan, Halifax.

Chauhan, Halifax, guidelines to evaluate changes in subjects will be forthcoming, including permutation analysis in which cut-offs for change for individual subjects will be derived.

Other imaging techniques, including scanning laser polarimetry and optical coherence tomography estimate the thickness of the retinal NFL in the area around the optic disc. Scanning laser polarimetry (Figure 7.6)

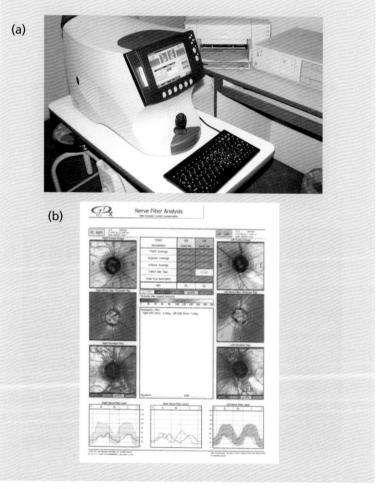

Figure 7.6 (a) The GDx nerve fiber layer analyzer and the (b) printout in a patient with glaucoma. The red and yellow dots in the printout show an abnormal nerve fiber layer (compared with normal) and suggest glaucoma.

estimates the thickness of the NFL by measuring retardation of polarized light by microtubules in the retinal NFL. It can also make estimates of change. As the NFL retards polarized light, retardation measurements are converted to NFL thickness values. The main limitation of this technology is that ocular structures other than the NFL retard polarized light and the degree of retardation may therefore vary in a manner unrelated to NFL thickness.

Optical coherence tomography (OCT) uses near-infrared light interferometry to identify cellular layers that differentially scatter light in the retina. Spectral domain OCT (SD-OCT) provides a sufficiently high resolution to map NFL thickness around the optic disc (Figure 7.7).

Programs to detect progression have been developed for both of these technologies, but depend on scan reliability and image registration.

Visual field examination. In terms of decision making, identifying functional defects is generally more important than finding structural changes. The 'Overview' and 'Glaucoma Progression Analysis (GPA)' programs on the Humphrey automated perimeter can be used to detect functional progression.

The Overview program takes a sequential series of visual field measurements over a period of time and displays them in a single printout (Figure 7.8). The printout contains all the information provided in the single field analysis, including total- and pattern-deviation plots (see Chapter 3, pages 57–9). Simple visual inspection of the Overview printout gives the physician a feel for stability or deterioration at a glance, and whether field deterioration is due to generalized sinking of the hill of vision or to glaucoma.

Worsening of the total-deviation plot alone usually indicates anterior-segment causes (cataract, refractive error, miosis, patient factors, etc.), and is rarely due to glaucoma. Persistent defects in the pattern-deviation plot indicate localized scotomas and suggest worsening of glaucoma.

The Overview printout tells a story and is a good 'first look'. It does not, however, provide the statistical help required to initiate changes in management, particularly surgical intervention. The GPA program provides such statistical help.

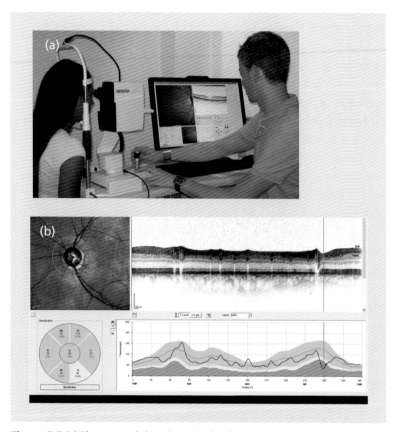

Figure 7.7 (a) The spectral domain optical coherence tomography machine. (b) Printout in a patient with glaucoma. The vertical green line shows a nerve fiber layer (NFL) defect. The thickness of the patient's NFL (black line) dips into the red (abnormal) area of the bottom graph at this point.

Glaucoma progression analysis. In the GPA program, the threshold value from the pattern-deviation plot of each test-point location in every follow-up field is compared with an average of threshold values from the same test point in two selected baseline fields. The GPA summary is incorporated into the single-field printout. If three or more points at any location in the field have worsened compared with the baseline on two consecutive tests, the GPA labels it as 'possible' progression. If three or more points at any location deteriorate in three consecutive tests, the program labels it as 'likely' progression (Figure 7.9).

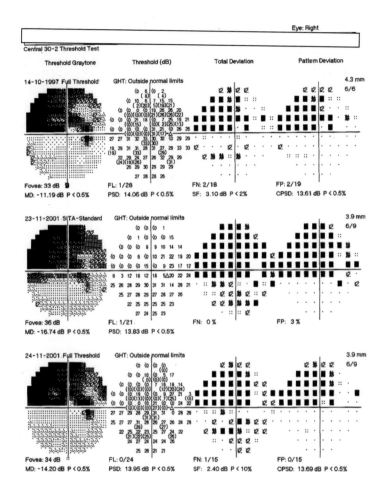

Figure 7.8 Overview program printout showing a sequential series of visual fields.

Unfortunately, the GPA program does not provide information on points that have improved. Clinically, any causes of false progression must be excluded. Selection of the baseline fields is particularly important and should not include 'learning curve' fields (see Figure 3.28, page 61). The baseline should be updated after any intervention for progression so that future changes can be detected.

The GPA uses the concept of event analysis to estimate whether today's field is worse than the baseline fields. It does not provide

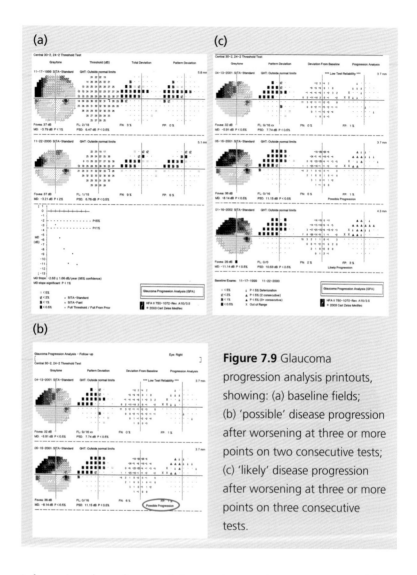

Figure 7.9 Glaucoma progression analysis printouts, showing: (a) baseline fields; (b) 'possible' disease progression after worsening at three or more points on two consecutive tests; (c) 'likely' disease progression after worsening at three or more points on three consecutive tests.

information about the rate of change, the most important aspect of the natural history of glaucoma. The only commercially available software that estimates point-wise progression (i.e. progression of a single visual field point) is 'Progressor' Windows PC software, which imports Humphrey visual field test data. It can perform point-wise linear progression and can produce a binocular visual field printout (Figure 7.10).

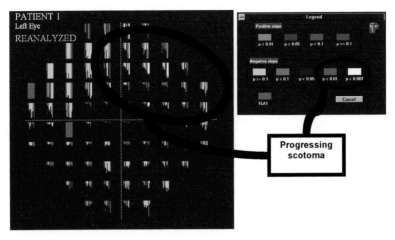

Figure 7.10 Point-wise linear progression performed by the Progressor software. Bar length indicates retinal sensitivity. Color indicates statistical certainty of the change.

Combining clinical signs with visual field test results. Retesting of visual field abnormalities significantly improves accuracy in recognizing disease progression. Randomized controlled trials typically require three or four confirmatory fields to confirm progression. In the clinic, however, the judgment of progression is more 'corroborative', taking into account other factors such as IOP (using several measurements over time at various times of the day), and appearance of the optic disc, NFL, hemorrhage, etc. If these factors suggest progression of glaucoma, then a first step could be a visual inspection ('eyeballing') of the overview printout to provide an idea of what is going on. This must be followed by examination of the GPA printout and/or the visual field index summary (see below). A label of 'possible' progression on the GPA printout corroborates clinical concern; a repeat field with a finding of 'likely' progression is then probably sufficient to take decisions, especially if the deteriorating points correlate with the optic disc findings.

The visual field index (VFI) is a new global index for the Humphrey Visual Field Analyzer used to determine progression. The VFI uses the pattern-deviation plot to provide an age-corrected visual field sensitivity

113

measure (this is minimally influenced by cataract). It is also 'center' weighted to better reflect the functional effect of ganglion cell loss and is calculated for all available reliable fields. The VFI is presented as a percentage of the full field (100% for normal function and 0% for perimetric blindness), and the rate of progression is displayed on a summary printout of the Humphrey perimeter. This summary printout shows two baseline fields (where the patient started) at the top, the rate of progression graph (the VFI) in the middle, and the most recent field (GPA analysis and alert) at the bottom. For the graph of rate of progression, the VFI is plotted against patient age and a linear regression slope is calculated when five or more fields are available. This represents the rate of progression in percentage loss per year and extrapolates the current rate of change up to 5 years.

Figure 7.11a shows the test results for an eye with clear visual field loss at baseline, with VFI values indicating that the remaining field is about 65% of a full field. The patient may be at risk of field loss during his lifetime, but the present rate of progression of -0.3 VFI% per year indicates that the field is relatively stable. When enough reliable data are available, an extrapolation of the current trend is performed to help predict what might happen in the future. In this case, the projected test result is expected to be almost the same as the current one.

Figure 7.11b shows the result for an eye with a smaller defect at baseline and a VFI of about 80%, but the rate of progression has been much faster. The patient has lost about 5 VFI% every year, and the VFI in her current field (after 7 years' follow-up) is 45%. If this trend is allowed to continue, the remaining field may be less than 20% in 5 years.

It is important to note that extrapolations provide only an indication of what might happen if current trends continue. Whether visual field progression is usually linear or whether the rate also varies over time is still debated. If those extrapolations suggest relative safety, as in Figure 7.11a, then the prudent course may well be to continue current therapy. However, if extrapolation suggests significant risk of visual disability, as in Figure 7.11b, then further intervention is required to slow the rate of progression to a safe and acceptable level. In all cases, however, the benefits of additional therapy must be weighed against the potential risks.

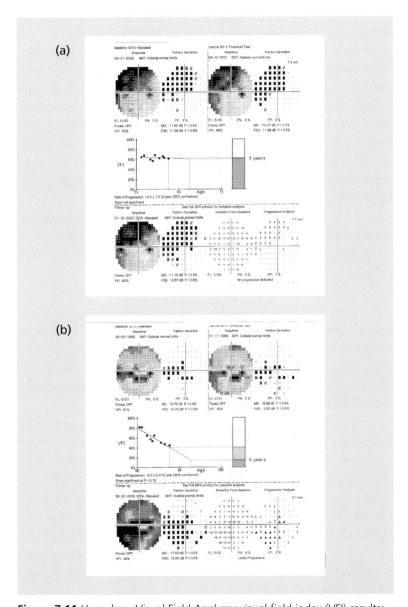

Figure 7.11 Humphrey Visual Field Analyzer visual field index (VFI) results: (a) Although there is clear visual field loss at baseline the VFI indicates that the field is relatively stable. (b) There is a smaller defect at baseline but the rate of progression is faster. (See text for details.) Reproduced courtesy of (a) Anders Heijl and (b) Boel Bengtsson, Malmo, Sweden.

Other forms of functional testing. Short wavelength automated perimetry (SWAP) can sometimes identify field defects when standard white-on-white automated perimetry (SAP) is normal. However, it is a difficult test to perform and is usually not part of routine clinical testing. Like SWAP, frequency doubling perimetry (FDP) and its variant Matrix can sometimes show glaucomatous defects when SAP is normal. Patients often find FDP easier than SAP, and FDP has undergone testing as a quick screening method for the detection of field defects from any cause. Change or progression analysis software are not available for either FDP or Matrix. Multifocal visual evoked potentials (mVEP) measure the amplitude (and latency) of brain waves generated from visual field stimulation. It has a role in glaucoma patients who are unable to perform subjective visual tests as well as in other optic nerve diseases.

Other tests. Routine measurement of blood pressure (BP) is desirable, as low ocular perfusion pressure (which is the difference between mean BP and IOP) is associated with increased risk of glaucoma progression. If glaucoma is progressing despite achieving the target IOP, referral to a physician to detect and avoid nocturnal 'dips' in BP is recommended. Exclusion of aggravating factors such as sleep apnea is also desirable. If the clinical course is atypical, the diagnosis should be reviewed and, if necessary, a neurological evaluation should be carried out.

Routine measurement of BP may also identify a patient with undiagnosed hypertension, just as glaucoma, diabetic retinopathy or cataract may be detected in patients during other routine medical examinations. Such 'case finding' circumvents some of the issues of population-based screening (see Chapter 8). It should also be borne in mind that sudden and drastic reductions in systemic BP must be avoided in a patient with glaucoma. Thus, management of hypertension in these patients requires particular care.

Key points – monitoring

- The patient with stable glaucoma requires 6–12-monthly follow-up. The frequency of follow-up visits must be individualized, and more examinations should be performed over a shorter period of time when any change in disease status is suspected.
- A comprehensive eye examination (or selected parts of it) and selected investigations should be performed at each follow-up visit. Baseline visual fields should be obtained for future comparisons.
- Progression of glaucoma is suspected from a combination of raised intraocular pressure and changes in the optic disc, nerve fiber layer or visual field.
- Structural changes can be confirmed by comparison of serial optic disc stereophotographs with the baseline findings, or by imaging techniques.
- Progression of a visual field defect is confirmed by the Visual Field Index (VFI) that incorporates the Glaucoma Progression Analysis (GPA) program. The VFI summary printout also provides an estimate of the rate of progression and uses this to extrapolate functional deterioration over the next 5 years.
- Findings from imaging and visual field evaluations should never be interpreted in isolation.

Glaucoma is the leading cause of irreversible blindness worldwide; the prevention of such morbidity should therefore be a priority. Some of the genes involved in congenital (*Cyp1B1*) and juvenile glaucoma (*GLC1A-GLC1J*) have been identified and it is now possible to test, identify and better manage those at high risk for these conditions. Predictive testing and genetic counseling are likely to play important roles in these scenarios.

However, we are a long way from undertaking similar testing for primary glaucoma in adults, especially for primary angle closure and primary angle-closure glaucoma (ACG), which cause such high morbidity. Although there are a number of candidate genes, they have been identified in only a small number of adults with primary glaucoma.

A strategy such as population-based (universal) screening or case detection (opportunistic screening) for the early identification of these blinding disorders is needed. With a condition as serious as glaucoma, it goes against the grain to wait for patients to come to us, when we can screen the population to detect disease at an earlier, perhaps more treatable, stage. Of course, implicit in this approach is the assumption that such screening provides more benefit than harm. This chapter examines the issue of screening the population for glaucoma and other prevention strategies. The example used is glaucoma, but the arguments are equally applicable to conditions such as diabetic retinopathy.

Criteria for universal (population-based) screening

The World Health Organization recommends that certain defined criteria be fulfilled before any population-based screening is undertaken (Table 8.1). Other questions also need to be asked before embarking on any screening program.

- Does early diagnosis lead to improved clinical outcomes in terms of visual function and quality of life?
- Can the health system cope with the additional clinical time and resources required to confirm the diagnosis and provide long-term care for those who screen positive?

TABLE 8.1

World Health Organization criteria for population-based screening

- The disease must be an important public health problem
- The disease must have a recognizable latent or early stage, during which individuals with the disease can be identified before symptoms develop
- An appropriate, acceptable and reasonably accurate screening test is available
- An accepted and effective treatment is available*
- The cost of case finding must be economically balanced in relation to possible expenditure on medical care as a whole

*The treatment must be more effective at preventing morbidity when initiated in the early asymptomatic stage than when begun in the late symptomatic stages of the disease.

- Is the incidental harm done by screening and by the information (correct or otherwise) small in relation to the total benefits from the screening–assessment–treatment system?
- Will the patients in whom early diagnosis is achieved comply with subsequent recommendations and treatment regimens?

It is important to remember that screening has to be an ongoing process, not a 'once and for all' project. This adds to the complexity.

Glaucoma fits some of the criteria required for screening, but others are more problematic; so, while the question of screening the population for glaucoma appears to be clear cut, the answer is not.

In order to evaluate the issue of universal screening (population-based detection) for glaucoma as a preventive measure, a number of terms need to be defined (Table 8.2). The predictive value of a test depends on the prevalence of glaucoma in the population being tested. As shown in Figure 8.1, assuming all other factors remain constant, the positive predictive value will rise with increasing prevalence. With a low prevalence of glaucoma, most of those positive test results will in fact be false positives unless the test is highly specific.

In order to increase the yield of the tests, the prevalence of glaucoma in the population must be reasonably high. The prevalence

TABLE 8.2

Definitions used in screening for glaucoma

Term	Definition
Universal (population-based) screening	Active risk assessment of the entire population (or everyone within a defined demographic group) to determine whether they are likely to have glaucoma, and to refer those that are for diagnostic evaluation
Case detection (opportunistic screening)	Active risk assessment for glaucoma when patients visit clinics and hospitals for other reasons. When this assessment is performed by an ophthalmologist, the diagnostic evaluation can proceed immediately where indicated.
Prevalence	The proportion of patients with glaucoma in the population tested at any given time
Sensitivity	The ability of a test to correctly identify individuals with glaucoma (true positives)
Specificity	The ability of a test to correctly identify individuals who do not have glaucoma (true negatives or normals)
Positive predictive value	The proportion of patients with positive test results who actually have glaucoma
Negative predictive value	The proportion of patients with negative test results who do not have glaucoma

of glaucoma can be 'increased' by targeting high-risk groups such as the elderly, individuals with a family history of glaucoma and patients with diabetes or myopia.

Tests used for screening

A test for glaucoma screening should have a reasonably high sensitivity with a very high specificity (see Box 3.1, page 31). A test with lower specificity will result in many false positives. Most glaucoma screening tests have lower specificity for earlier stages of the disease. Prevent Blindness America recommends 95–98% specificity and 85% sensitivity

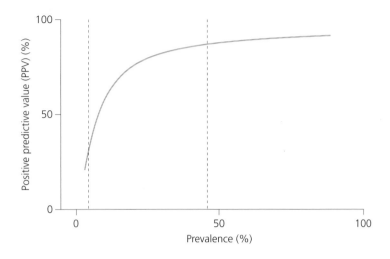

Figure 8.1 Relationship between positive predictive value and prevalence.

for moderate-to-severe glaucoma. For screening purposes, it may be better to target the moderate and advanced cases that require more urgent treatment. Diagnostic tests will also have a higher sensitivity and specificity in such cases.

The tests for screening/case detection are discussed below. Details of specific diagnostic tests are given in Chapter 3.

Primary open-angle glaucoma (OAG).

Measurement of intraocular pressure. Tonometry has a poor sensitivity and specificity for manifest glaucoma. For the detection of primary OAG, at a cut-off of at least 21 mmHg, tonometry has a poor sensitivity (47.1%) and specificity (92.4%), so the rules of 'SpPIN' and 'SnNOUT' (see Box 3.1, page 31) cannot be applied. Half of all patients with primary OAG have intraocular pressure (IOP) below 22 mmHg at a single screening. Furthermore, many individuals with a raised IOP may never develop optic nerve damage. IOP measurement alone is therefore an inefficient tool to screen populations for glaucoma.

Assessment of visual field. The gold standard in perimetry is conventional white-on-white automated perimetry, which has a good sensitivity (97%) but poor specificity (84%). However, it is still a time-consuming and laborious screening device, despite improvements in testing strategies.

Frequency doubling perimetry (FDP) is an alternative to standard visual field testing and can rapidly detect established field defects. FDP has been reported to have a sensitivity of 55% and a specificity of 92% when used in a population-based sample.

Examination of the optic disc and nerve fiber layer (NFL). The sensitivity and specificity of evaluation of the optic disc depend on the technique used and the diagnostic criteria for glaucoma. Using a cup-to-disc ratio of 0.55 as a cut-off, the sensitivity is 59% and the specificity 73%. Inter-observer agreement on optic disc examination by clinical methods or fundus photographs is very high in some centers and poor in others.

Newer imaging techniques for the optic disc and NFL are promising, but are expensive and have not been validated. The small numbers of studies performed have shown various combinations of disc parameters, IOP and family history to have only moderate sensitivity (49–66%) and specificity (79–87%) for glaucoma.

Combined scoring algorithms. The best screening test reported to date uses a combination of signs and risk factors to establish a likelihood score. Depending on the cut-off value selected, sensitivities and specificities of 89.9% and 98.1% have been reported.

Primary angle-closure glaucoma. Population-based studies in the West have shown that the prevalence of OAG is five times that of primary ACG. Primary ACG is more common in the Asian region and half the glaucoma blindness in the world is estimated to be due to angle closure. In order to be effective, any screening/case detection initiative has to include methods to detect angle closure.

Primary angle closure (PAC) can occur without raised IOP or optic disc/visual field changes. That is the best stage to detect the disease.

Tonometry will only detect PAC in individuals with a raised IOP.

Structural and functional tests, as described above for OAG (optic disc examination, perimetry etc.) will only detect primary ACG that has damaged the optic disc or visual field. However, approximately 75% of subjects with primary ACG in Asia have optic nerve damage, and screening strategies that detect functional damage in primary OAG may also be suitable for primary ACG. Such tests will not identify eyes without functional damage, nor eyes at risk for angle closure.

Gonioscopy. The ideal way to identify angle closure and eyes at risk of angle closure is to examine the angle using a gonioscope, but the clinical expertise and instrumentation required render gonioscopy inappropriate for screening.

Anterior chamber depth/axial length ratio. Methods to identify eyes at risk of angle closure include assessment of the anterior chamber depth, as well as the anterior chamber depth to axial length ratio. However, the sensitivity and specificity of these techniques do not make them appropriate for screening. Furthermore, they require expensive instrumentation and trained technicians.

Flashlight and van Herick tests. In the flashlight test (sensitivity 80–86%, specificity 69–70%), a light is shone from the temporal side of the eye onto the cornea, parallel but anterior to the iris. A shadow on the nasal limbus identifies an eye with a shallow anterior chamber at risk of closure. The van Herick test (sensitivity 61.9%, specificity 89.3%) uses a slit beam to compare the depth of the peripheral anterior chamber with the thickness of the cornea.

It is important to remember that these two tests only detect occludable angles, which are a risk factor for angle closure; they do not detect angle closure. This distinction is important because only a minority of occludable angles progress to angle closure. Using the van Herick test for screening would result in too many false positives, and the flashlight test is worse in this respect.

It is possible to obtain a higher specificity (or sensitivity) by using tests in combination. If the van Herick test is positive and the IOP is raised, the specificity improves to 99.3% but the sensitivity will decrease. As far as a population-based screening strategy is concerned, this combined specificity is high enough to actually treat the patient as having angle closure.

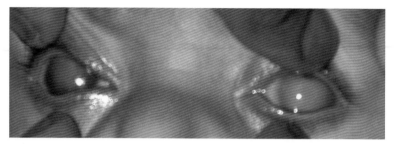

Figure 8.2 Child with congenital glaucoma with characteristic hazy corneas.

Primary congenital glaucoma. In addition to raised IOP, signs of congenital glaucoma include a large corneal diameter (see page 64) and a hazy cornea (Figure 8.2). All health professionals responsible for newborn babies should be able to identify these signs and immediately refer the patient to a specialist. The same is true for any infant or child complaining of photophobia and/or watering of the eyes.

As children all over the world are immunized against a variety of diseases, all pediatricians and caregivers responsible for providing immunization should be familiar with such obvious signs of ocular pathology. This will help with early detection and treatment of congenital glaucoma and other potentially blinding, even life-threatening, conditions such as retinoblastoma.

Problems with universal screening

The arguments below apply even when high-risk groups like the elderly or residents of homes for the elderly are targeted for screening.

Obligation to the patient. When a patient comes to the clinic they are seeking help; we treat them to the best of our ability but without a guarantee for cure. In screening, we are seeking the patient, which implies that we are going to make them better. When we seek out patients we are obliged to establish a diagnosis and treat those who have glaucoma. If we do not have the appropriate infrastructure to establish diagnosis and provide treatment, then screening is not justified. Some countries may not have the requisite infrastructure to follow up and categorize those individuals who test positive, or even to treat them appropriately.

Glaucoma management, both medical and surgical, is intensive. In this situation, it is perhaps inappropriate to screen the entire population. Also, we must remember that, in order to be effective, such screening cannot be a one-off event; even developed countries may not be able to afford to screen the population at large for glaucoma and handle the burden of further testing, treatment and follow-up.

Specialist techniques. Diagnosis of glaucoma requires state-of-the-art techniques, as detailed in Chapters 3 and 7. Certainly, the presence of glaucoma cannot be confirmed using only screening techniques.

False positives and negatives. A false-positive test result risks burdening the patient with the disease label, which can have severe consequences. For example, normal children misdiagnosed as having heart disease become as handicapped as children who have the disease. In fact, because of the number of false positives, the amount of disability from cardiac 'non-disease' greatly exceeds that from actual heart disease. Similarly, delivering a diagnosis of glaucoma or suspicion of glaucoma has many psychological implications.

Finally, patients who actually have the disease but test negative are given a clean bill of health, which may discourage future screening and thus appropriate diagnosis and treatment.

Case detection (opportunistic screening)

In contrast to universal screening, case detection relies on detection of disease (glaucoma) only in patients who are visiting a health clinic for another reason.

Most elderly patients, people with myopia or diabetes (all at risk for glaucoma), visit ophthalmologists and optometrists for other eyecare needs. They also visit physicians for their medical needs. The prevalence of glaucoma is higher in these individuals and as such most of the tests described above – tonometry, ophthalmoscopy and perimetry – have a high positive predictive value. Gonioscopy is the gold standard for the diagnosis of primary ACG.

The general physician also has an important role in the diagnosis of OAG; ophthalmoscopy and FDP can both be performed in a physician's

> **Key points – prevention**
>
> - Predictive genetic testing, genetic counseling and follow-up of individuals at high risk are possible for congenital and juvenile glaucoma but not for adult primary glaucoma.
> - Population-based screening is not a viable strategy for glaucoma.
> - Diagnosis of glaucoma should rely on case detection when patients present to clinics for other complaints.
> - A comprehensive eye examination for all those who visit an ophthalmologist or other eyecare professional is the only way to reliably detect glaucoma.

office (just as the measurement of blood pressure to detect hypertension is feasible in the ophthalmologist's office).

Recommendations

Universal screening is not recommended at present because the cost–benefit ratio is uncertain. In addition, universal screening is not feasible for developing countries that do not have an adequate infrastructure in terms of the availability of expertise (trained ophthalmologists), time and instrumentation to confirm the diagnosis among individuals who test positive. Adequate infrastructure also means the availability of expertise (trained surgeons) and instrumentation to treat those in whom the diagnosis is confirmed. (The word 'feasible' in this context refers to modern preferred practice.)

Each country will need to make a decision on population-based screening based on an assessment of the ground reality. While some more developed countries may opt to target high-risk groups for universal screening, this would be a distant objective in most developing nations.

Case detection. To effectively detect glaucoma, any person over the age of 35 years who seeks ophthalmic attention for any reason should have a comprehensive eye examination, as described in Chapter 3, including the tests listed in Table 8.3.

Gonioscopy is mandatory for any person suspected of having glaucoma, irrespective of whether the suspicion is based on a raised IOP, changes in the optic disc or visual field defects.

The World Glaucoma Association consensus meeting concluded that the flashlight and/or van Herick tests (see above) are not appropriate tools to diagnose angle closure. A positive flashlight or van Herick test requires confirmation by gonioscopy. Van Herrick assessment combined with IOP measurement may have a role in screening.

TABLE 8.3

Tests to detect glaucoma in a comprehensive eye examination

Tonometry
Ideal: applanation tonometry
Less than ideal: pneumotonometry or Schiotz tonometry

Slit-lamp biomicroscopy

Gonioscopy
Ideal: indentation gonioscopy using a Sussman, Zeiss or Posner lens
Acceptable: Goldmann single- or two-mirror lens with 'manipulation'
Some patients cannot tolerate an indentation examination and others cannot tolerate a Goldmann lens; it is probably desirable to have both types of gonioscopes available

Dilated evaluation of the optic disc
Ideal: dilated stereoscopic evaluation by slit-lamp biomicroscopy; fundus photography
Acceptable: direct ophthalmoscopy

Visual field examination
Ideal: a full threshold test using calibrated white-on-white automated perimetry, or Goldmann perimetry performed by a trained technician
Acceptable: frequency doubling perimetry, or a Bjerrum screen (used by a trained experienced person)
If the IOP is > 21 mmHg and/or the disc shows 'suspicious' changes, the patient should undergo a visual field examination.

Note: the tests are not listed in the order they may be performed.

Useful resources

American Glaucoma Society
Tel: +1 415 561 8587
ags@aao.org
www.glaucomaweb.org

Association of Optometrists (UK)
Tel: +44 (0)20 7261 9661
www.aop.org.uk

European Glaucoma Society
www.eugs.org

The Glaucoma Foundation (USA)
Tel: +1 212 285 0080
info@glaucomafoundation.org
www.glaucomafoundation.org

Glaucoma and Ocular
Hypertension Patient Advocacy
Center (GLOHPAC)
http://glohpac.proboards.com

Glaucoma Research Foundation
(USA)
Toll-free: 1 800 826 6693
Tel: +1 415 986 3162
question@glaucoma.org
www.glaucoma.org

Glaucoma Service Foundation to
Prevent Blindness (USA)
Tel: +1 215 928 3283
www.willsglaucoma.org

International Glaucoma
Association
SightLine: +44 (0)1233 64 81 70
Tel: +44 (0)1233 64 81 64
info@iga.org.uk
www.glaucoma-association.com

Prevent Blindness America
Toll-free: 1 800 331 2020
www.preventblindness.org

South East Asia Glaucoma
Interest Group (SEAGIG)
info@seagig.org
www.seagig.org

World Glaucoma Association
Tel: +31 20 679 3411
info@worldglaucoma.org
www.worldglaucoma.org

World Glaucoma Patient
Association (WGPA)
www.worldgpa.org

Further reading

The AGIS Investigators. The Advanced Glaucoma Intervention Study (AGIS): 7. The relationship between control of intraocular pressure and visual field deterioration. *Am J Ophthalmol* 2000;130:429–40.

Chauhan BC, Garway-Heath DF, Goni FJ et al. Practical recommendations for measuring rates of visual field change in glaucoma. *Br J Ophthalmol* 2008;92:569–73.

Hong C, Yamamoto T, eds. *Angle Closure Glaucoma*. Kugler Publications, 2007.

Kass MA, Heuer DK, Higginbotham EJ et al. The Ocular Hypertension Treatment Study: a randomized trial determines that topical ocular hypotensive medication delays or prevents the onset of primary open-angle glaucoma. *Arch Ophthalmol* 2002;120:701–13.

Leske MC, Heijl A, Hyman L et al. Predictors of long-term progression in the Early Manifest Glaucoma Trial. *Ophthalmology* 2007;114:1965–72.

NICE Clinical Guideline 85. *Management of chronic open angle glaucoma and ocular hypertension*. London: National Collaborating Centre for Acute Care, 2009. www.nice.org.uk/nicemedia/pdf/CG85 FullGuideline.pdf

Parikh RS, Parikh SR, Navin S et al. Practical approach to medical management of glaucoma. *Indian J Ophthalmol* 2008;56:223–30.

Parrish RK, Feuer WJ, Schiffman JC et al. Five-year follow-up optic disc findings of the Collaborative Initial Glaucoma Treatment Study. *Am J Ophthalmol* 2009;147:717–24.

Quigley HA, Broman AT. The number of people with glaucoma worldwide in 2010 and 2020. *Br J Ophthalmol* 2006;90:262–7.

SEAGIG *Asia Pacific Glaucoma Guidelines*. Sydney: South East Asia Glaucoma Interest Group, 2003–4. www.seagig.org/toc/APGGuidelines NMview.pdf

Shaarawy TM, Sherwood MB, Hitchings RA, Crowston JG, eds. *Glaucoma. Vol 1: Medical Diagnosis and Therapy*. Elsevier, 2009.

Stamper RL, Lieberman MF, Drake MV, eds. *Becker–Shaffer's Diagnosis and Therapy of the Glaucomas*. 8th edn. Mosby, 2009.

Thomas R, Sekhar GC, Parikh R. Primary angle closure glaucoma: a developing world perspective. *Clin Experiment Ophthalmol* 2007;35:374–8.

Trope GE, ed. *Glaucoma Surgery*. Informa Healthcare, 2005.

Index